Revisioning Phenomenology:
Nursing and Health Science Research

Revisioning Phenomenology:
Nursing and Health Science Research

Patricia L. Munhall, ARNP, Ed.D., PsyA, FAAN
Associate Dean of Graduate Program
Director of the Center for Nursing Science
School of Nursing
Barry University
Miami, Florida

National League for Nursing Press • New York
Pub. No. 41-2545

The views expressed in this book reflect those of the authors
and do not necessarily reflect the official views of the National
League for Nursing.

Library of Congress Cataloging-in-Publication Data

Munhall, Patricia L.
    Revisioning phenomenology: Nursing and health science
research / Patricia L. Munhall
        p. cm.
    Includes index and bibliographical references.
    ISBN 0-88737-597-9 : $37.95
    1. Nursing—Research. 2. Phenomenology. I. Title.
RT81.5.M855 1994
610.73'072—dc20   94-1454
                                                              CIP

This book was set in Garamond by Publications Development Company, Crockett, Texas.
The editor and designer was Allan Graubard. The printer was Clarkwood Corp. The cover
was designed by Lauren Stevens.

Printed in the United States of America.

To all those who have and continue to search for meaning.

*Any meaning is better
than none at all.*
NIETZSCHE

Contents

Preface
Green Leaves, Sour Grapes, and Writing for Mirabella

G ail Sheehy has written another number one best seller. This one, called *The Silent Passage,* has a fresh green leaf on the cover, and the critics' blurbs within tout it to be revolutionary. Gail Sheehy has discovered menopause and second to that has brought it out of the closet. This literary feat was, to some extent, autobiographical and self-motivated, but that is beside the point.

In Sheehy's introduction, she lists all the people she consulted to produce her work. Among them is every conceivable scientist or health professional but a nurse. A nurse is among the women interviewed who apparently don't know a thing about menopause.

FREELY CROSSED DISCIPLINES

Here is the author's list of her "freely crossed disciplines": She reached "beyond the obvious medical practitioners"—gynecologists, breast surgeons, and internists—to "endocrinologists, . . . research physiologists, neuroscientists, psychologists, psychiatrists, and gerontologists" also "nutritionists and Chinese medicine doctors" (p. ix). To enlarge her scope of knowledge, Sheehy also consulted "scholars in sociology, anthropology, historians, and primate researchers" (p. x). That nurse researchers were not among her scholars does not mean, however, that nurses did not make it into this volume at all.

THE NURSE INTERVIEWEE

Among the more than one hundred women in various stages of menopause whom Sheehy interviewed, there was a nurse; this is how she is quoted:

> *My mother had a surgical menopause in her early forties,"* mentioned *Gloria, a nurse from an Italian American family, "so I really don't know much about it." (p. 28)*

Then *it* becomes worse. Gloria began to have symptoms, and so members of the group asked her if she had seen a doctor. Her response: "'No' admitted the nurse. 'I was going to coax myself out of it, be calm, take deep breaths'" (p. 28).

Though the narrative goes on to share that Gloria almost lost her job because of her menopausal symptoms (or lack of knowledge about them), nurses in this book are not entirely without value. The Nurses' Health Study is used for vital statistics about heart disease, broken bones, and estrogen therapy. What irony that nurses should be the sample for a physician's group study of women!

NURSE RESEARCHERS AND MENOPAUSE

It is glaringly obvious that Sheehy did not consult one of the many nurse researchers who have devoted much research to gain understanding and knowledge about the phenomenon of menopause. To me, it is abominable that the critical work of nurse researchers in this area was not cited—not only because nursing research deserves recognition but also because that knowledge *was* researched in scientific ways that deserve the public's attention.

LESSONS TO BE LEARNED

There are lessons here for us as nurse researchers. First, Sheehy's study is not restrictively method bound. She is primarily a journalist who went out and asked, "What's it like to experience menopause?" or "What is the meaning of menopause?" She used all sorts of data from existential life worlds: the temporal, the spatial, the corporeal, and the relational. She calls it research, but she does it with freedom. This is liberating even though it limits scientific scholarliness. As a journalist, however, she does look for "Truth."

Sheehy does not label her research phenomenological or ethnographic, but who cannot recognize this attribute when reading the book with the green leaf of life on the cover? Strict methodologists would be quick to label this work pop psychology. Indeed, the depiction of the California group of women did resemble Mary McCarthy's version of *The Group* grown older more than it resembled a focus group for research.

Second, her interpretation might lead to cynicism. The upbeat idea of "beginning" a second adulthood is quite appealing; as if we could be 13 years old again! There's something Sheehy did with numbers that makes it so. Though to some readers that may seem silly, it is preferable to the mechanistic view of menopause as a process of deteriorating, wearing out, and losing value.

MAINSTREAMING

However, the lessons: Obviously, our research needs to find a place in mainstream literature, and to do that, the research must be written in a conversational, informative style, not unlike Sheehy's approach. Also, we must not be so rigidly bound by methods that require us to ask questions of form rather than substance. How are we to discover new methods if we cannot go beyond the boundaries of the old?

How many of us as doctoral student advisors or researchers would have let a study on menopause or any other phenomenon be so free, imaginative, and dramatic? How many of us have a book on the best seller list about a major life process that is within nursing's research domain? I don't, and I regret that my doctoral students who have completed important dissertations don't. We were only following methods.

MAGAZINE DISPLAY

Running, Nike, Freedom, Just Do It! Going public into mainstream magazines or what might be called popular literature (though that may be construed by some as an oxymoron) is essential for the public and the profession alike. Just so—many nurse editors and authors have proposed this transition.

I am putting forth this proposal: Let those of us who plan to write an article this year write that article for the public. Let's not be silent, and next year, let's come back here with our list of publications. Let's forget sour grapes and send off our green leaves to *Mirabella* and the like thereof. Let nurses be recognized as authorities. Same time, same place, next year. Let's make a lot of noise.

The foregoing text was submitted to a prestigious journal to be considered for publication; I received the following letter in response:

Dear Dr. Munhall:

Thank you for submitting your manuscript entitled, "Green Leaves, Sour Grapes, and Writing for Mirabella." I regret to inform you that it has not been accepted for publication.

While I agree with everything you had to say, the paper reads like a position paper or editorial. Since you are not an editor, you cannot write editorials.

That piece is good and I want to keep it in my drawer of good ideas and thoughts, so you might find some of the ideas in the journal's editorial.

Thank you for considering us.

Sincerely,
Editor

I have included my article here as a way of introducing the many meanings of study from a phenomenological perspective.

This book is designed from that point of view. It provides examples of experiences that are human, giving meaning to living and hope for a more compassionate world.

PATRICIA L. MUNHALL

Prologue

T his work is an attempt to write about phenomenology from a phenomenological perspective. In many ways, therefore, the book is a phenomenology of the meaning of studying some "thing" and, in this presentation, keeps reflecting back on itself. This reflection is "real," grounded in the things themselves and in material that I hope restores the lifeblood to research. Barthes (1986) states:

> *Some people speak of method greedily, demandingly; what they want in work is method; to them it never seems rigorous enough, formal enough. Method becomes a law . . . the invariable fact is that a work which constantly proclaims its will-to-method is ultimately sterile: everything has been put into the method, nothing remains for the writing; the researcher insists that his texts will be methodological, but this text never comes: no surer way to kill a piece of research and send it to join the great scrap heap of abandoned projects than Method.*

This book is not to be construed as antimethod. In fact, I acknowledge a situated context in the world at this time. The icons of research—method, hypothesis, and proof—belong to the age of modernism. We are not about to abandon these sacred beliefs even though the age of modernism is said to be dead.

Phenomenology, I believe, because it entered our lives as researchers in a time that still could be construed as modern, developed its own icons. The university thrives on tradition and upholding cherished beliefs and ways of being. Thus, phenomenological "methods" brought acceptance and confidence to those doing such study and also to those guiding such study.

We are now in a "post" era, and as in any post era, remnants of the previous era very much influence what we do. This work attempts to satisfy that era while urging us to consider how we come "to know" in what has been variously called the postindustrial, postmodern, postpatriarchy, or poststructural era.

Universities, which are still structurally oriented, produce social scientists educated as method idolators. I have borrowed the following example from Postman's (1992) study of social science research results published in the *New York Times:*

1. December 5, 1989—"Recent research findings have discovered that people fear death."
2. September 11, 1990—"Results of new research which suggests that Asian-American students do well in school because they come from families that value advanced academic degrees."
3. October 2, 1990—Research has "reported that psychologists have discovered that children who are inept at social relations tend to be unpopular with other children."

These examples illustrate two contextual areas of research. First, method-driven students are very much with us, regardless of the epistemological or ontological value of their work; second, some human scientists are questioning meaning and being, and are probing, going underneath, and behind what appears and what is concealed.

Critical to this latter group are human scientists who are tugging at phenomenology to fit into a method that would be considered scientific. And then there are those human scientists who recognize the disorganization, discontinuity, and diversity of anything "living." Instead of yielding to oversimplification, they accept ambiguity and uncertainty, follow impulses, respect intuition, await appearances, and above all revere the stories that humans tell of their being in the world. They have learned to listen, accept silence, be patient, assume "unknowing," give up cherished beliefs, and realize that their research is fulfilled in writing, as described in the Preface of this book.

If we are indeed in a transition from one age to another, then it is necessary to address both method and phenomenology. In this volume, you will come upon traditional formats as well as ways of "doing" a study from a phenomenological perspective and—material about phenomenology. From a postmodern perspective, this work attempts to decrease the distance between the reader and the writer. Also, I want the reader to experience the book, not just read it. As a demonstration of the phenomenological perspective, the book itself illustrates the composition of a piece of phenomenological writing.

This book is about the meaning of being human. Being-in-the-world, being here, being there, being present, coming into being are all viewpoints within these pages. There is structural being; and there is creative being. I prefer to think of phenomenology as the study of being, which offers itself to study in experience. Thus at the outset, the structural concept of phenomenology is the study of lived experience and is sometimes referred to as such within this work. This approach is hardly possible, however, without acknowledging that we are studying human beings experiencing something or being something.

A more precise conceptualization of the phenomenological perspective resides here: It is the study of being human. What does it mean to be a human being? This premodern idea transcends temporality and assumes its place of eminence in the postmodern age. Choosing how "to be" with your study will be a matter of assessing your situated context. There are no value judgments per se (how can an author escape that susceptibility?), and if you are new to the phenomenological perspective, the structure in Chapter 1 and Appendexes B, E, and F, will undoubtedly be helpful. Hundreds of students have said that their thesis or dissertation was well accepted when presented in this structured form.

This is understandable since the structure preserves tradition. I wonder how a university committee would react if a student presented *The Silent Passage: A Study of Menopause,* as it is presently written. Now here is something you might find odd. I encourage any student who is pursuing a qualitative method to follow a structured format. I believe it is essential for students to come to understand the meaning of phenomenology as a whole by learning to recognize its essential components. In terms of *The Silent Passage,* I probably would have some difficulty with it from a methodological perspective, which also reveals that I have a lot more growing to do myself. Although that is my situated context, my perspective is to liberate us from preconceptions. If we were spoon-fed preconceptions from another era, the icons prevalent in that era remain stubbornly present. The reader may find examples of that, and may even experience my "modern age" way of being, and my struggle to meet the challenge of becoming part of the postmodern time that is at hand.

At hand is also the desire of many students to study "meaning." Just as phenomenology was once thought of as a reaction to logical positivism, this search for meaning today may be a response to the advance of technology, the changes in power structures, the vacuum left by a discredited materialism, and the need to balance scientism with compassion, care, and understanding.

In many ways, this book is a conversation. I would like for you to think of it as friendly, and I have minimized abstraction to reduce the distance between the reader and text. I also introduce my own friends and experiences, as well as the experiences of students and colleagues.

I hope you are moved by some of the writings about "being" in experience. At the time of their happening, people laughed, cried, and supported one another. They began to understand the *other*—to understand meaning.

I have been most fortunate in having opportunities for such experiences with students and colleagues, to be a part of a process where intellectual barriers to expression are dropped and we all become with each other. Sometimes I reflect, "What really went on in those classes?" We learned more, I suppose, about the process of phenomenological study. Yet, in doing just that, I believe we fulfilled an aim of such study; we became more human.

I hope this will be your experience as well.

Acknowledgments

I wish to thank my students, some of whose writings appear in this book. In their own search for meaning, they have moved me deeply: Pat Hurst, Monique Biondolillo, Lauren Barlow, Brenda Blanchette, Susan Manter, Vivian Sanchez, Vivian Moore, Joanne Masella, Robin Petit, Tomas Madayag, Maribel Mezquita, Sandra Bagaley, Robin Parker, and Dan Little.

I also wish to thank colleagues who have joined in their own ways to attach significance to the matter of meaning and thus have contributed to my own search. Among them are Zane Robinson Wolfe, Suzanne Langer, and Carol Germain where, during a 1992 summer workshop, a volume on women's experience (soon to be published) was conceived. Sarah Lauterbach joins in that volume, and I thank her for being first an ideal student and now a colleague. This also can be said for Lucy Warren, whose study appears in this book. Also appreciation needs to be expressed to Carolyn Oiler Boyd, who first showed me perceptual differences in coming to know. The works of Max van Manen have thoroughly influenced my thinking, and I am so grateful for his humanness.

Chuck, in this book, is Charles Beauchamp, RN PhD, Chair of the Department of Nursing, at Colby-Sawyer in New Hampshire, and Ray is Raymond Klimasewski, a special education teacher. I thank them both for their friendship and support, as well as their permission to tell about our experiences. The inclusion of their perspective in the text is deeply appreciated.

I go on because of meaning, so I want to thank my sons, Dennis and Craig, for providing me with all sorts of lived experiences that continue to give my life extraordinary meaning.

A special thank you to three people who are part of this effort: Maureen Rock, who patiently deciphered my handwriting and who said to me one day, "You know, you're doing in this book exactly what you're writing about"; her wonderful mother, Audrey MacCormack, who generously assisted her; and Allan Graubard, my editor, whose wisdom and support of projects are so deeply appreciated.

I would also like to extend my appreciation to Dr. Judith Balcerski, Dean of the School of Nursing, and Karol Geimer, my secretary, for their warmth and support. Also, to Jean Watson, a thank-you for being a constant source of inspiration; and to Virginia Fitzsimons, a thank-you for being what the word friend really means.

This work is the work of many people. In this new age, all I can aim for is to make a modest contribution that encourages appreciation of others, values the meaning of being human, and looks toward a "being" that is meaningful.

Dancing to the Beat of a Different Drum
Horizontal Perception

This chapter combines anecdotal material with a background or horizon that places phenomenology within the present situated context.

The chapter discusses perception and then the philosophical underpinnings of qualitative and phenomenological research. It also alludes to the meaning of loss that can be felt when least expected, if you are mindful, awake, and reflective. These three critical ways of being in experience, are thus used as examples of being-in-the-world.

Along with this introductory material, the reader might also read Appendixes A, E, and F. This material has to do with beginning to understand phenomenology as a perspective. Elsewhere, this understanding is referred to as a stream or current of thinking. Dance softly. *

---

* Parts of this discussion come from P. L. Munhall's "Philosophical Ponderings on Qualitative Research," and "Qualitative Research Methods" in Brink and Woods *Advanced Methods for Nursing Research*. Reprinted with permission from Chestnut House Publishing and Sage Publications respectively.

A RIDE TO THE AIRPORT

I was driving my friends, Chuck and Ray, to the airport in Miami one Friday morning, engaging in small talk as people are inclined to do on such a short drive. I had arisen earlier than usual to pick them up, and when I arrived at their place—five minutes from mine—they were not ready. I did not complain: in fact, I joked with them and overall "acted" like a good friend. I was, however, somewhat aware of being irritated; I knew I was tired and that the tiredness was going to affect me the rest of the day. Thoughts were in my head as to why they hadn't called a taxi, for surely they would have if I wasn't nearby, and taking a taxi was not a financial problem. Also, since they were my close friends, I never was thrilled when they left town.

As we drove toward the airport, I casually said something, of no particular consequence (I thought) to Chuck. He replied, "Why are you being so nasty?" To which, I immediately snapped back, "I'm not being nasty—or didn't mean to be nasty." A few moments elapsed, and I realized something quite simple. I then apologized to Chuck and said, "You know, it's not important whether what I said was nasty but that you perceived it as such."

Afterward I thought to myself how odd: I, as a student, teacher, and researcher, had long been a writer about perception, subjectivity, and unknowing; and yet, it was in that moment I understood, in my soul, the meaning of perception.

In fact, I first taught a course in phenomenology five years ago. Since then I've taught other courses, seminars, and workshops on this philosophy, perspective, or approach. It took five years to come to this kind of personal understanding. This is not to say I did not "know" about perception or understand perception before. As both a nurse and psychoanalyst, perception has always been center stage for me. What I do know now, from this experience, is that there is a coming to know at a deeper level, and it can catch you up short and, most importantly, override previous learning or perception. I will call such moments of insight "breaking a cognitive barrier" because they go so deep—I now not only know but *feel* and am changed. I have experienced an affective and emotive change of knowing in addition to my more ordinary cognitive knowing.

Phenomenology, the subject of this book, is a philosophy, an approach, or perspective to living, learning, and doing research. Many disciplines that believe themselves to be wholly, if not partly, a human science have made an interpretive turn toward a phenomenologically oriented perspective.

"Lived experience" is often the phrase that becomes the focus of phenomenology. By now, many of us are familiar with the phenomenological imperative: "To the things themselves," attributed to Husserl. Thus a ride to the airport reflects this; a new interpretation is evolving and being reflected upon. We will return to this moment. Also, the phenomenological perspective begs us to look at ordinary daily human life experiences in their context to discover meaning. In that way, we can search without preconceptions in our efforts to better understand:

- Our being.
- Our being-in-the-world.
- What it means to be human.
- Where being is in life worlds.
- The verbal meaning of the words "human" and "being."
- The process of becoming, of achieving greater humanness.

In my living phenomenologically, which is what I struggle to do, I understand, at once, my situated context: I am an American woman living in the last decade of the twentieth century. I have transcended my first marriage and have two grown children, following their own mythologies of being. I work as both a professor of nursing and a psychoanalyst in contexts where all sorts of myths, rituals, beliefs, and perceptions are played out. Like you (to allow for an assumption), I interact with friends, neighbors, relatives, and various other humans who have their life histories, present-day life worlds, and individual meanings of events and objects. When I really understand that I cannot make assumptions about any of these people, or anything, then I can be phenomenologically present to them.

THE HORIZON FOR NURSING AND THE HUMAN SCIENCES

At this point, it is necessary to properly situate this work in the context of its cognitive "background" or horizon. Afterward, I will return to the emphasis that phenomenologists, or perhaps human beings thinking from that perspective, place on ordinary day-to-day experiences of life. It is the taken-for-grantedness, the sailing-through-life without reflection, the dazed going-through-the-motions learned from whatever context that give way too often to the meaninglessness and alienation so characteristic of our situated context in the postmodern age. Phenomenology, as a way of being, takes us from this dazed perspective to a gazed perspective where we give, reflect, and attempt to understand the "whatness" of ordinary life. When connotations of the word "ordinary" turn on negative possibilities as they seem to, the need for the phenomenological gaze becomes more apparent. In a sequential thought process, ordinary life seems negative, void of meaning. Allowing for reflection on the ordinary, however, can lead to extraordinary understandings, for example, my penetrating moment while driving my friends to the Miami airport.

An Interpretive Turn

For some years now, nurse theorists and human science researchers have engaged in a lively and enlightening critique of the positivism, empiricist, and mechanistic assumptions on which much of nursing knowledge has evolved (see Baer, 1979; Benoliel, 1984; Chinn, 1985; Davis, 1973; Hutchinson, 1986; Leininger, 1985; Lidemann, 1979; MacPherson, 1983; Meleis, 1985; Moccia, 1986a, 1986b; Newman, 1979, 1983; Norris, 1982; Oiler, 1982; Oiler-Boyd, 1993; Omery 1983; Parse, 1987; Coyne & Smith, 1985; Paterson & Zderad, 1976; Silva, 1977; Stern, 1980; Swanson & Chenitz, 1982, 1986; Watson, 1981; and others). Many who initiated what was to become an "interpretive turn" in nursing research began to think of nursing as a human science, different from the natural sciences such as chemistry and biology. With that "turn" came an increased interest and exploration into research methods that differed from the traditional scientific method and were more congruent with a specifically human science. These research methods, although highly differentiated, have been grouped together into a "qualitative" scheme to contrast them conceptually with "quantitative" methods. In this work, quantitative methods are associated with positivistic assumptions about reality, while qualitative methods are associated with assumptions or philosophical underpinnings of phenomenology. I'll begin, as I have, with the question of perception.

A Question of Perception

In March the Gypsies returned. This time they brought a telescope and a magnifying glass the size of a drum, which they exhibited as the latest discovery of the Jews of Amsterdam. They placed a Gypsy woman at one end of the village and set up the telescope at the entrance to the tent. For the price of five reales, people could look into the telescope and see the Gypsy woman an arm's length away. "Science has eliminated distance," Melguaides proclaimed.

Gabriel García Márquez
One Hundred Years of Solitude, (1970, p. 12)

Was Melguaides correct in this assertion? Some might say no, since distance as objective reality still did exist. Yet the appearance of distance, the perception of distance, was eliminated. Thus we have an example of a reality independent of the telescopic observer and of a reality that includes the observer. However, it is important to note that superimposed in the first instance is contemporary knowledge about distance. Readers today might even enjoy this novel conclusion to the discovery of magnification. Nevertheless, from the perspective of the philosophical underpinnings of qualitative research, at the moment in time depicted by García Márquez, the experienced reality was an expression of consciousness, a human perspective of the world. The appearance of the specific phenomenon and the perceived world was the reality. Oiler (1986b) emphasizes this:

This is not to be confused with truth. As access to truth, perception presents us with evidence of the world not as it is thought, but as it is lived. Perception of an amputated limb as an ambivalent presence is not truth but it is reality. (p. 87)

As with the perception of distance, individuals choose reality by assigning meaning to the objective world. The subjective experience and the objective world, within this conceptualization, are inseparable; they are one.

In health care practice, this inseparability is manifested every day and often with astounding confirmation of the preceding premise. For example, a patient manifests specific objective data for a nurse to attend to and make a judgment. What will matter in this situation is, first, the patient's perception of the objective data and, second, the nurse's response to the patient's action. As shown by the following statements about the same phenomenon, a patient may perceive data in many different ways:

- "Should I call the nurse?"
- "It's probably nothing; I'll let it go."
- "This could be serious; I'll wait and see and call the nurse if it continues."
- "This is serious; I'd better call the nurse immediately."

Different perceptions will lead to different actions as the patient responds to such thoughts. In this patient's case, different nurses may also have different responses. Again, perception is what will define reality. The nurse may perceive:

- This patient needs reassurance.
- This patient needs medication.
- This patient is entering a threatening phase and bears watching.
- This is an emergency.

With each set of data rises the possibility of interactive perceptual responses. Reality then is defined by the perceptions of the patient and of the nurse. The nurse and patient assign meaning to the situation based on their own experience, history, and social customs. Without context, the data merely exist; for the situation to have meaning, the participants must perceive it in a certain way. In this example again, the world of a measurable or observable entity and the activity of consciousness merge. Without consciousness, it would seem, then that nothing matters. Without perception, we would think nothing.

A Question of Philosophy

Sarter (1988a) states that philosophy "is inquiry into the nature of reality through rational or intuitive thought" (p. 4). The traditional goal of philosophy is wisdom and the understanding of "truth." Health care professionals are concerned with some fundamental questions about the nature of human beings, the nature of the environment, and the interaction between the two. What we believe about health, illness, and nursing is derived from what we believe about the nature of reality. Furthermore, the research within the discipline is influenced by its belief system, worldview, or ideology. This worldview will contain assumptions that guide the research process and should reflect congruence between the philosophical system of the discipline and the research questions asked.

A Question of Nursing and Human Science Philosophy

Nursing and other human sciences have identified themselves as humanistic professions; they adhere to a basic philosophy that focuses on individuality and the belief that the actions of individuals are in some sense free. Free will is grounded in a worldview that sees the individual acting on experience. The individual chooses and is self-determined; in essence, the individual is an active being. Inherent to humanism are philosophical beliefs and values found within human science philosophies and expressed in such language as becoming, freedom, self-determination, autonomy, advocacy, and human potential (Munhall, 1982). A belief in holism is predictably stated and posits that a human being's integration does not allow an investigator to know an individual by breaking the person into parts and piecing them back together. Often within nursing philosophies, nurses speak of the individual as a system that is open, evolving, and emerging in mutual interaction with the environment. Also, individual uniqueness is valued and spoken about in

terms of culture, socioeconomic, religious, and experiential rela-
tivism. With such a holistic view of the individual—unique and self-
determined—it is understood that each person experiences his or
her own "reality." Although the experience may be shared, the individual remains final arbiter, who interprets and gives meaning to
the experience.

Some nursing philosophies situate the nurse as advocate of the patient's autonomy and as acting to safeguard the patient's rights.
Curtin (1979) suggests that this advocacy is the philosophical foundation of nursing. Watson (1985) has been clear about her philosophical commitments; human beings are nonreducible experiencing subjects characterized by freedom, choice, and responsibility. Health is a
process; there is an interconnected evolution of the human and the
world and an epistemology for nursing should allow for aesthetics,
ethics, intuition, and process discovery. Other nursing theories exemplify similar philosophical assumptions although distinctions
among them can be found.

In this regard, Sarter (1988b) analyzes of the philosophical roots of
four contemporary nursing theories—Rogers' (1970) science of unitary human beings, Newman's (1986) theory of expanding consciousness, Watson's (1985) theory of human care, and Parse's (1981) theory of man-living-health and urges nurses to establish a coherent and
common philosophical foundation and orientation. Other human sciences, such as psychology, sociology, and (dare I say) some schools of
medicine, struggle as well with this quest for humanistic ideals, reflective of worldview or paradigm that expresses caring and reverence for being human.

On Qualitative Research Methods in General

Before proceeding with the discussion of philosophical underpinnings of qualitative research, it may be helpful to take a look at how
some nurse theorists and researchers perceive these methods. In addition, the language as expressed by these writers links the language of many stated nursing philosophies with the philosophical
underpinnings of the method. The significance of language here is
its liberating or constraining qualities as well as its revelatory

inescapability. It is the experience and use of such language that lays open, either implicitly or explicitly, assumptions, beliefs, values, and priorities.

The general description of qualitative methods in research, as noted earlier, is part of the horizon or background that phenomenology (as an approach) has been umbrellaed under. Although this idea is quite prevalent, it remains somewhat paradoxical, for phenomenology may be the real underpinning of qualitative methods. However, to stay within the situated context, what follows is an acceptable sequence in the description of phenomenology.

Benoliel (1984), for example, explains qualitative research methods

> *as modes of systematic inquiry concerned with understanding human beings and the nature of their transactions with themselves and with their surroundings. (p. 3)*

and goes on:

> *Qualitative approaches in science are distinct modes of inquiry oriented toward understanding the unique nature of human thoughts, behaviors, negotiations, and institutions under different sets of historical and environment circumstances. (p. 7)*

Leininger (1985) offers this concretion:

> *The qualitative type of research refers to the methods and techniques of observing, documentating, interpreting attributes, patterns, characteristics, and meanings of specific, contextual, or gestaltic features of phenomena under study. (p. 5)*

Wilson (1985) points to the nonquantitative aspects of qualitative research and states:

> *Qualitative analysis is the nonnumerical organization and interpretation of data in order to discover patterns, themes, forms, and qualities found in field notes, interview transcripts, open-ended questionnaires, journals, and diaries. (p. 397)*

Field and Morse (1985) write:

> *Qualitative methods should be used when there is little known*
> *about a domain, when the investigator suspects that the present*
> *knowledge or theories may be biased or when the research question*
> *pertains to understanding or describing a particular phenomenon*
> *or event about which little is known. (p. 11)*

At present, the most prevalent qualitative research approaches used by nurses and human science researchers are phenomenology, grounded theory, ethnography, history, case studies, and analytic philosophy. Discussions of these methods can be found in textbooks by Leininger (1985), Field and Morse (1985), Munhall and Oiler (1986, 1993), Parse et al., (1985), Swanson and Chenitz (1986), and perhaps others in press at this writing.

On Philosophical Underpinnings of Qualitative Research

The philosophical underpinnings of qualitative research methods reflect beliefs, values, and assumptions about the nature of human beings, the nature of the environment, and the interaction between the two. Researchers doing qualitative research perceive reality and assign meaning to their efforts from the perspective of some of the following assumptions:

- Individuals are viewed within an open perspective as active agents, interpreting their own experience and creating themselves by their inner existential choices.
- Individuals and specific groups of individuals have varying histories, varying "here and nows," and varying perceptions of the "future."
- The world and its people are constantly changing and evolving: This assumes a dynamic realty.
- "Truth" is an interpretation of some phenomenon: The more shared that interpretation is, the more factual it seems to be, yet it remains temporal and cultural. Exploration may be "partially

true" depending on certain variable conditions and then only "true" for specific individuals.

- Interacting with subjects does not mean the suspension of "objects." Objectivity, itself, can be viewed as a subjective discovery, a perception on its own.
- The subjective experience of the individual or group is valued and described. Meaning comes from the source and is not presumed, assumed, or assigned.
- Linguistic, social, and cultural considerations help imbue experience with meaning.

Ethical Assumptions of Qualitative Research Methods

Although it is difficult to ferret out ethical assumptions from the philosophical underpinnings of qualitative research in general, the following list presents several factors that seem particularly relevant in the exploratory designs of qualitative research methods.

- Human beings are as they are. There is no preplanned effort to change individuals or groups with a qualitative method. Effort is toward discovery and understanding of experience.
- Actions of individuals are in some sense free. They are free to be as they are (naturalistic).
- There is a reverence for the human experience de nova, the descriptions of which contribute to the ability to understand and be empathic. Such fresh understandings may be the impetus for further theory development, intervention, and social change.
- Researchers do not predetermine reality through their own assumptions and language. The research subjects are the authors of their biographies and experiences.

In summary, the ethical assumptions of qualitative methods spring from a reverence for the subjective, self-determined, self-described realities of individuals and groups (Punch, 1986; Munhall, 1988). Phenomenology is one such approach that actualizes this potential.

ON PARADIGMS, PHILOSOPHIES, AND THE PROLIFERATION OF BOTH

The philosophical underpinnings of qualitative research methods could be said to represent a paradigm or research tradition. Kuhn (1970) suggests that a paradigm is a discipline's specific method of solving a puzzle, of viewing human experience, and of structuring reality. The influence of a paradigm cannot be overstated since it structures the questions to be asked while *systematically eliminating* those kinds of questions that cannot be stated within the concepts and tools of a specific paradigm. Laudan (1977) writes about a similar concept, renaming it a research tradition, and states:

> *A research tradition is a set of general assumptions about the entities and process in a domain study and about the appropriate methods to be used for investigating the problems and constructing the theories in that domain. (p. 81)*

A paradigm that many nurse researchers believe deserving of consideration is what the German philosopher Wilhelm Dilthey (1926) called the *Geisteswissenchaften* or human sciences. According to Dilthey, the human sciences are to be distinguished from the natural sciences because of critical and fundamental differences in attitude toward their respective phenomena of research. Stated simply, the natural sciences investigate objects *from the outside to the inside,* whereas the human sciences depend on a perspective *from the inside to the outside.* The most important concern in the human sciences is that of *meaning.* Meaning exists within human subjectivity rather than material nature. Thus, the aims of the two sciences are different. The natural sciences seek *causal explanation, prediction, and control.* The human sciences seek *understanding and interpretation.*

The Empirical-Analytical Paradigm

In the empirical-analytical paradigm—natural science—an important assumption specifies that the world is structured by lawlike generalities that can be identified, predicted, manipulated, and controlled. Observation and measurement yield universal statements for scientific theory. The world is ordered and understandable in an objective sense, and there is the belief that the knower can be differentiated from the known. Reality is reduced to the measurable and the empirical, and is stated in terms of dependent and independent variables. The basic worldview is mechanistic; in it, humans are seen to react in a prescribed manner to specific stimuli. Because mathematics is usually essential to theory construction here, methods are derived from quantitative models as well as being referred to as empirical and positivistic. The empirical-analytical paradigm attempts to present a formalized account of the nature of scientific knowledge that will enable prediction and control, words that are not necessarily pejorative. Indeed, nurses need theory, knowledge of relationships, and identified interventions to help predict and control human responses to specific situations.

However, this knowledge, when and if applied, is not always sufficient. There are many other considerations in the world of human life experiences. While microorganisms in a laboratory test tube might be thought to be under control, in the human environmental field, they might be out of that context of control. In the human life world, microorganisms usually become more obstinate and opportunistic than in a laboratory. Indeed, they can seem "out of control" when compared with their behavior under laboratory conditions. Simply, mice in a cage and pigeons in a laboratory are not the same as embodied human beings experiencing the social, cultural, and historical world. Not all that is real can be seen or measured. What is important to our understanding from a paradigmatic perspective, however, is that the exclusive use of any approach to science would systematically eliminate those kinds of questions that cannot be stated within the concepts and tools of one paradigm. Therefore, it would be to a discipline's advantage to be open and encouraging of multiple paradigms.

The early history of nursing and health care research derives its traditions from the empiric-analytic approach. From 1964 to 1976, there was unequivocal commitment to this worldview (Abdellah, 1969; Dickoff & James, 1968; Hardy, 1974; Jacox, 1974). Silva and Rothbart (1984), however, identify 1976 as the year in which nursing and health care research began to question this commitment. Questions began to rise about the adequacy of strictly quantitative research methods to test nursing theory deductions. At this time, as well, alternative approaches to empiricism began to appear in the literature. These approaches were sought for the possibilities they offered for understanding phenomena that are not necessarily material, observable, and measurable. Phenomenology, a philosophy and research approach believed to be consistent with human science assumptions, was one of these research approaches.

The Phenomenological Paradigm

As an alternative and a historical reaction to the then prevailing hegemony of the positivist perspective, phenomenology construed itself as a philosophy, a perspective, and an approach to practice and research. Philosophically, phenomenology seems to undergird many of the qualitative research approaches (although some argue this point). Because of its importance as a philosophy, some key concepts are presented here. Recognition needs to be given to Husserl who introduced the idea of phenomenology in response to or in reaction to the context-free generalizations of the positivist approach of the natural sciences. Husserl attempted to restore the "reality" of humans in their "life worlds," to capture the "meaning" of this, and to revive philosophy with new humanism. Spiegelberg (1976), Cohen (1987), and Reeder (1987) provide excellent discussions of the history of the phenomenological movement. These concepts then, as outlined, reflect an acknowledgment of the inevitability of subjectivity in any exploration or description of reality. This inevitability is not stated with resignation but with the idea that subjectivity expands and enriches the authenticity of perceptions and understandings of phenomenona. It is this perspective that is both essential and desirable.

Key Concepts of Phenomenology as Philosophy

As defined by Merleau-Ponty (1962–1964), *consciousness* is sensory awareness of and response to the environment. Consciousness is life: It is not an interior or inner existence, it is existence in the world through the body. The unity of mind and body becomes a means of experiencing, thus eliminating the idea of a subjective and objective world. A person cannot step out of consciousness and be sure of anything. The world is knowable only through the subjectivity of being in the world. Objectivity as a quest for reliability and validity depends on the recognition of this relationship between mind and body, subject and object, and the knowledge that this or any knowing comes about through consciousness.

Embodiment explains that through consciousness we are aware of being-in-the world, and it is through the body that we gain access to this world. We feel, think, taste, touch, hear, and are conscious through the opportunities the body offers. There is talk sometimes about expanding the mind or expanding waistlines. The expansion is within the body, within consciousness. At any point in time and for each individual, a particular perspective or consciousness exists based on the individual's history, knowledge of the world, and perhaps openness to the world. Human science's focus on the individual and on the meaning events may have for an individual reflects the recognition that experience is individually interpreted.

The *natural attitude* (Schutz, 1970) is a mode of consciousness that espouses interpreted experiences. The world as experienced and interpreted by preceding generations is handed down, teaching a great deal about reality in the process. These teachings become assumptions, unquestioned meanings about phenomena, that are a part of a person's "natural attitude" toward the world. To hear or see something contrary to the natural attitude can be disconcerting. This attitude of being in the world is deeply ingrained and usually unquestioned. Understanding the concept of natural attitude can help in understanding, at the individual level, the responses to change. Both the perspectival and the physiological alterations associated with a life change are often the result of a *disruption* of the natural attitude.

Experience and *perception* are our original modes of consciousness. Perception, which takes place through the body, is an individual's access to experience in the world. Perception of varying objects depends also on the context in which they are experienced for interpretation and meaning. A person who says the aim of phenomenology is to describe lived experience may be describing his or her own or another's perceptions of that lived experience.

Perception of experience is what matters, not what in reality may appear to be contrary or more "truthful." If a person perceives danger when "in fact" there may be none, in the reality of that person's lived experience, there *is* danger. Perhaps that is why saying "this won't hurt" or "this will only hurt for a little while" is often ineffective in allaying a person's fear. The perception of the lived experience may not even be of pain; the perception may be of a danger far worse than being hurt or feeling pain. Interpretation of the experience from the individual's unique perception of an event is critical. What is important from this worldview, therefore, is not what is happening but what is perceived as happening. That is the reality to be concerned with—the experience as the individual is perceiving it.

As a philosophy, phenomenology demonstrates these major concepts in the many interpretations that exist concerning its meaning. A phenomenological question here might be asked: "What it is like to try to understand phenomenology?" or "What makes someone think and talk about phenomenology?" The answers are found in the themes of consciousness, embodiment, the natural attitude, perception, and experience. Again, these two questions would be good grist for the phenomenological perspective as a qualitative approach to research.

Phenomenology as Philosophy: More Key Concepts

The relational view of the person posited by Heidegger (1927) further elaborates on the philosophical theme of phenomenology. Because an individual participates in cultural, social, and historical contexts of the world, to be human is to "be-in-the-world." Language, cultural, and social practices are handed down to individuals who embody the meanings and interpretations of these practices. In Heideggerian phenomenology, the interpretation and self-understanding handed down through language and culture are called the "background" (Allen, Benner, & Diekelmann, 1986). The idea of the background (like the natural attitude) is critical because it provides conditions for human actions and perceptions. It is where the individual is, a history to the present moment, and a view of "what can be."

Other Heideggerian ideas include:

- Meaning is found in the transaction between an individual and a situation so that the individual both constitutes and is constituted by the situation.

- Human purposes and concerns "prestructure" the human world so that what is considered significant about an event or object is a function of or embodies that concern (Dreyfus, 1972). The perception of meaning follows from this understanding.
- This understanding is predicated on the belief that immediate experience is embodied with organization and meaning, with linguistic, social, and cultural patterning, and with characteristics intrinsic to the experience.
- A critical assumption of this phenomenological perspective is its emphasis on language, which imbues and informs experience. Language does not exist apart from thought or perception, for language generates and constrains the human life world.

Key Concepts of Phenomenology as Research

Max van Manen (1984) has offered the following observations about phenomenological research:

- Phenomenology is the study of the individual's life world, as experienced rather than as conceptualized, categorized, or theorized. Phenomenology aims for a deeper understanding of the nature or meaning of everyday experiences.
- Phenomenological research is the study of essences of experience. In phenomenology, the researcher does not ask, "How do nursing students learn to nurse?" but asks instead "What is the nature of the experience of becoming a nurse?" The aim is to understand the experience. The opportunities for plausible insights bring the investigator in more direct contact with the world.
- Phenomenological research is the attentive practice of thoughtfulness—a minding, a heeding, a caring attunement, a wondering about the project of living. When the language of a lived experience awakens a person to the meaning of the experience, he or she gains a fuller understanding of what it means to be human.
- Phenomenological research is a quest for what it means to be human. The more deeply a person understands human experience,

the more fully and uniquely he or she becomes human. Such individuals learn to notice and to make sense of the various aspects of human existence. Of course, the more often a person engages in such attentiveness, the more he or she should be able to understand the details as well as the more global dimensions of life. The corollary is that such previously unreflected upon phenomena, the "taken for granted," assume richer meaningfulness.

• Phenomenology has been called "the science of examples." Phenomenological descriptions are often composed of examples that permit readers "to see" the deeper significance or structure of the lived experience being described.

Other phenomenologists include but are not limited to Georgi (1970), van Kaam (1969), and Colaizzi (1978). (See Appendix A.) Additionally, paradigms that have similarities and yet distinctive differences from the preceding approaches—and also contribute to the philosophical underpinnings of qualitative research—include but are not limited to critical social theory (Allen, 1985), evolutionary idealism (Sarter, 1988a), feminism (MacPherson, 1983; Chinn, 1985), simultaneity (Parse, 1987), a reflective mode (Crowling, 1986), and historicism (Laudan, 1977).

With the proliferation of philosophical paradigms being discussed by nurse and human science scholars, it is important to study critically the underlying assumptions that frame these different modes of inquiry. According to Morgan (1983), "Assumptions make messes researchable, often at the cost of great oversimplication and in a way that is highly problematic" (p. 377).

On Assumptions

Assumptions or philosophical underpinnings of a research method become, to some degree, part of the constructed knowledge; the investigators' assumptions about reality underpin their research studies. Assumptions then can become self-justifying and self-fulfilling approaches to deal with the diversity of competing points of view. Morgan (1983) discusses supremacy, that is, rank ordering by truth value, to determine the merits of assumptions. Morgan also uses synthesis to enable an integration, capitalizing on strengths and minimizing weaknesses of differences between and among assumptions. Contingency judges assumptions according to their usefulness. Dialectic attempts to use the differences among competing perspectives for constructing new modes of understanding. Finally, Morgan cites Feyerabend as an advocate of epistemological "anarchism" in science. Simply put, Feyerabend states: "that there is no idea, however ancient or absurd, that is not capable of improving our knowledge" (p. 380).

Feyerabend is committed to a creative humanism that asks this question: *Is there a contradiction between creativity and method?*

Of these five approaches—supremacy, synthesis, contingency, dialectic, anarchism—nursing literature favors the dialectic (Moccia, 1986a, 1986b), which is founded on assumptions that provide a worldview similar to certain nursing perspectives. Furthermore, the dialectic offers an alternative to struggling between and among methods; instead, this approach rephrases choice as a searching for internal relationships between and among methods. In this regard, Meleis (1986) has outlined both what she believes is the major domain of assumptions and the paradoxes that a dialectic approach can help researchers understand and solve. Among these paradoxes are particularism and holism, uniqueness and generalization, and genderless, or nonsexist, theories.

When discussing the philosophical underpinning of qualitative methods (as in this book), it is critical to attend to assumptions. The significance of assumptions was recognized by Kuhn (1970) insofar as paradigms are built on the very assumptions that have the potential of *defining* a worldview and are deemed important and possible to study.

From Philosophical Underpinnings to Praxis

Interest in qualitative research is directed toward the fulfilling of a humanistic, existential, phenomenological philosophy. With the phenomena of concern to nurses being human responses (American Nurses Association, 1980), the researcher becomes oriented toward discovering and uncovering insights, meanings, and understanding of those responses. I substitute here "experiences" for "responses" and assume a phenomenological perspective. Nursing and human sciences are interested in the nature of language, the interaction of human beings with cultural, social, and historical inevitabilities and experiences. Viewing existence as dynamic, we seek to understand and interpret the meaning of "being" in experience.

At this juncture, it is appropriate to transverse the course from named abstractions of philosophical underpinnings to praxis: the concrete. This section, then, provides continued assumptions about qualitative research (and, therefore, phenomenology) along with discussion of some practical reasons for pursuing qualitative research.

In research, a person or situation presents interests, problems, or questions that the researcher can often respond to in one of two general ways: The researcher can respond from extrapolation and hunches about what is known or assumed about the phenomenon or can suspend preconceptions or inferences and say: "I'm not sure about that"; "I don't know about that"; "There's virtually nothing known about that." The first response lends itself to traditional hypothesis testing and deduction from existing theory; the second response lends itself to research activities such as "going out," "finding out," or asking "what's going on here," and leads to understanding theory development.

Consider an easy example of method as derived from traditional hypothesis testing and deduction from existing theory. The context is a question: "What is it like being married?" A deductive approach would initially require a return to the literature on marriage and family to arrive at workable hunches. These hunches would then allow the researcher to link variables found in the literature to marriage. From the linking of variables, hypotheses would arise. These hypotheses would provide direction for the study and might include the following dependent variables: increased role stress, role conflict, or role ambiguity. Marriage, of course, might increase life satisfaction, sense of generativity, or decrease interaction with old friends. The answer to the question—"What is it like being married?"—would be primarily based on what can be deduced from what is already known.

In contrast, this same question—"What is it like being married?"—can be answered from a qualitative perspective. This is particularly appropriate when there is an interest in the *meaning* of the lived experience of being married. In a qualitative study, answers may be obtained by asking people the study question in a direct way or by spending time observing and interacting with people who are married. Interviewing people, observing people, and, perhaps, in this case, asking people to keep diaries or other written material would all yield fresh authentic data. Questions that lend themselves to qualitative methods start with:

"What's going on here?"
"How does it feel to be _____?"
"What's it like to be _____?"
"What does this mean?"

With qualitative study, the researcher is seeking to discover knowledge or seeking to develop or formulate theory from the authentic source by looking at the whole within the social, the experiential, the linguistic, and cultural contexts.

Qualitative methods are further directed toward discovering or uncovering new insights, meaning, and understandings. Qualitative research is often serendipitous, leads often to wonderment, and requires from researchers a certain flexibility. Consider here other points of praxis within qualitative methods from a phenomenological perspective:

- There may be a current theory about the subject a reseacher wishes to investigate; however, that which is known may now be out of contemporary context. Answers to the question—"What is it like being married?"—differ dramatically from one generation to another. Descriptions and theories need to be revised in light of societal changes, other discoveries, and human evolution. Knowledge is culturally and time bounded. As culture "advances" and time "progresses," different descriptions and explanations are critical to understanding the meaning of different experiences.

- The philosophy advanced by nursing embraces the whole of the human condition with values that include respect for each individual and that individual's cultural interpretation of meaning in experience and events. Thus, there is an emphasis on self-determination and autonomy. In this regard, the phenomenological perspective becomes essential for nursing research as well as for the actual implementation of a holistic, empathic, individualized delivery of care. When the investigator asks, "What is the lived experience of being married about?" this implies an exploratory, open, theory-suspended approach actualizing the belief that the individual interprets his or her own experiences and gives meaning to them.

- With qualitative research, there is an attempted suspension or bracketing out of what the researcher has already come to believe, suspect, or assume. Qualitative designs yield new understanding and insights. Qualitative research can help emancipate the researcher from personal preconceptions of reality.

- Qualitative research studies are needed in current theory formulation and reformulation to access the extent to which biases have influenced worldviews and have established norms and standards that may be inappropriately generalized.

Some phenomenological philosophical underpinnings of qualitative research have been explored and discussed within the scope of this section for introductory aims. The assumptions that have been presented here need to be explored, argued about, examined for contradictions (because they are there), and disagreed with. The complexities and ambiguities in life as in research cannot be discounted. Nor should such complexities and ambiguities stimulate a yearning for the material, the measurable, the given.

Some researchers and practitioners will accept the challenge to ferret out meanings, glean insights, and understand the excitement associated with discovery. In a meaningful way, that is what phenomenology is all about.

MY TODAY

I can now look back on much of the previous text and understand: Because of my American education, I learned to write and think in that manner. As a reader and a writer (like many of you who are also writers), this is all part of my situated context.

The human sciences in this country and elsewhere struggle with a paradox. By keeping science as a discipline, some detachment is always present. But detachment, while championed by the scientific method, is itself complex and ambiguous. Certainly, it guarantees little beyond its own claims. In this regard, detachment is problematic to the researcher, the writer, and the reader. Unfortunately, the writing beginning with the section of this chapter called "An Interpretive Turn" reveals this problematic.

Yet what of human philosophy? Must human values, beliefs, and meanings be scientized even in the name of phenomenology? When reading philosophy, the reader enters an internal dialogue that involves struggling through entanglements, puzzles, and contradictions. But then, as I have previously stated, such problems may be in the nature of the contemporary phenomena under investigation. Thus, I have purposely situated this book as a demonstration of the academic and the world of meaning, both in terms of phenomenology. I also assume that many readers will desire a "how-to-do." To help such readers, and to enhance the cognitive and academic usefulness of the book, I will provide the "how-to-do" it. Even so, the how-to-do-it information resounds in the experience itself, the experience being always more vital.

As I write, the text talks to me, challenges me to think. The text of your study should do the same. Steps, however, imply a linear process not congruent with phenomenology. Living seems at least more circular than linear, and so in thinking and doing phenomenology the researcher enters a way of being. That way of being is different because we are accustomed to talking *to* or *about* the experience, not talking *in* or *with* the experience. Here, phenomenology calls upon us to do the following:

- Listen to the experience.
- Feel the experience.
- Be unknowing.
- Become with the experience.
- Raise our consciousness: the ordinary now becomes wondrous and extraordinary.
- Feel amazed.
- Feel puzzled.
- Begin to understand differences as "real."

Here circular, reflective, or spontaneous moments exist side by side. Although most phenomenologists speak of consciousness, often in a study the material of the unconscious is raised and slips into consciousness. Individuals will say "I never realized that before," and you most likely will experience that yourself.

BACK TO THE AIRPORT TRIP

In this first chapter, I will not "perform" a hermeneutic analysis of the airport experience in philosophical terms. Yet, my airport trip has a much deeper meaning than I assign to it, and discerning that meaning is the role of the phenomenologist who may be nurse, teacher, or therapist.

Whether or not nastiness on my part was there, as accused, Chuck brought it up as a possible way that I was "being." At a superficial glance, that could be true—they should have set their alarm clock earlier; they should have been ready when I arrived; they should have called a cab. A person might say that I was justified in being nasty.

Of course, this is not entirely the point. Hidden, and not too deeply either is that all phenomenology starts out with the personal. I was going through the lived experience of being abandoned. How many of us on last days with loved ones, before they go, or we go (because does it matter who goes?) have experiences fringed with emotions of hurt or anger? Because we often reexperience earlier events through the immediate, conversing about and reflecting on an ordinary experience can bring deeper understanding. Separating from those we care about or who care about us—an ordinary, sometimes daily, experience—is pungent with meaning.

For philosophers and scientists, such pungency reveals being. In terms of meaning, however, the scientist will often see only the symptom. So as human science researchers, we may come upon the manifestations of living out abandonment or sympathy in assessing the symptoms of anger, depression, headaches, digestive disorders, interpersonal conflicts, and on and on. What is behind the presenting symptom? What is concealed behind the appearance? There is an appearance—a showing of a phenomenon—that we may study provided we are aware of possibilities of disguise. Something becomes known that was not known earlier. In taking the world as it appears, we can—through the understanding of individual perception—come upon the *misunderstood*. We realize that *meaning was hidden within the appearance.*

This scenario, as a way of being, is beautifully captured by Miller (1993), when her main character, Lottie, during a funeral:

> *fumbles in her purse for a Kleenex . . . Ryan [her son] grabs her arm momentarily in sympathy* assuming, *Lotti* supposes, *that she's weeping for Jessica. Let him, she thinks. Soon enough he'll learn that you can mourn for any loss at any funeral; that there comes to be a general sense of sorrow and loss in life which can be released by the ceremony even of someone you didn't know. (p. 245)*

And that concludes the anecdote of the airport trip. Or does it?

2

Sitting on the Dock All Day Contemplating Myself Away
Phenomenology Taking Up Residence

In this chapter we dwell with some ideas within context that may take up residence in our being and what it means to be human. Also in this chapter, I disclaim originality of the ideas presented here. The ideas are a synthesis of experience and I remain a student. However, this idea of the meaning of being is unquestionably an extraordinary question and offered in this chapter are some tentative ways one might pursue this ponderous puzzle of life. Language and existential investigaton are proposed as means of engagement.

I'm sitting in my office at the university and a student is excited about her research proposal. This is not unusual, and the dialogue goes something like this:

Student: I've decided to study the lived experience of receiving nursing care by homeless women.

Me: How come?

Student: I'm interested in nursing as it relates to homeless women.

Me: (Should know better, but ask) Why not study the experience of being homeless for women?

Student: I think that's important but right now I want to study the nursing end.

The context of my "being" in this situation for a good length of time has taught me not to, nor should I, dissuade students from their own interests. Whatever choices they make, learning should take place in some way. So for both students and faculty members, a true phenomenological study should not get bogged down at the level of determining the phenomenon to be studied. Phenomenology should not be normative. The students and I are in different existential lifeworlds; I will respect theirs. This can be difficult, but is part of the educational process.

Me: Go ahead then. How do you intend to proceed?

Student: I don't know how many interviews I have to do. Is six enough? I'm not sure what bracketing is. How long should the interview be?

Me: If you are using phenomenology as an approach, there are no answers until you start. You will find the direction for your study by immersing yourself in the phenomenon.

Student: But what about the method?

Me: Phenomenology as a philosophical perspective is perhaps difficult to understand. However, there is no "method." "Bracketing" is not sacred, if even possible. Phenomenology is not ten transcribed interviews. It is not extracting themes. It is an approach to understanding human beings, what happens to them and what meaning these events or experiences holds for them. Each quest for understanding should be guided by the unfolding of the material that speaks language pertinent to your research. It's as though you are on a path, and every time you finish something on that path it will help you decide where to go next; you can take two roads or more. Just be sure that you are aware of what you are doing and why you are doing it.

Student: (somewhat frustrated) I really need to know how to do this. I've read studies that said they were phenomenological

but they sounded so scientific, meaning units, structural definitions. They didn't seem to grasp me. Is that the way it's
done?

Me: I'm teaching a course this spring on the phenomenological
perspective. I think its unrealistic to think that students can do
such work without a foundation. Perhaps you will enroll in it
and we can concomitantly work on your thesis.

Thus developed courses, Saturday seminars, and summer workshops. I have indeed learned and am still questing; meanwhile, I
hope that students also have come to understandings that will help
them progress. At this juncture, I am attempting to place the "thus
far" in writing. A book emerges.

This book should contain material for conversation about the way
the philosophy of phenomenology guides many research projects in
human science fields. Much of the inspiration for the suggestions
herein originates in the "everydayness" of my being. The entity of
being is integrated with many other entities, including researcher
and professor. All this takes place in time, some of which is past,
some of which is now, and some of which lies ahead. Existence in
this world, place, and time with others poses for me more questions
than answers. Searching for meaning continues without conclusion.
I find myself always probing deeper for understanding. Once I think
I understand something, I am already thinking about alternative understandings, especially, what might be concealed in this particular
understanding.

This work acknowledges what Heidegger said:

*Thus the term phenomenology expresses a maxim which can be for-
mulated as "to the things themselves." It is opposed to all free floating constructions and accidental findings; it is opposed to taking
over any conceptions which only seem to be demonstrated; it is opposed to those questions which parade themselves as "problems" often for generations at a time. (p. 30)*

I do not want to characterize "a problem." I wish to suggest a
worldview that is open and fluid to the study of humans being and
what it means to be human.

However, before embarking on this text, I did consider what was being done under the rubric of phenomenology, and those considerations have guided the development of the ideas presented here. Therefore, this book was not written without presuppositions and you may recognize them as personal to me as you go through the text. Some of you may share them and others will not. What I have to say within this book did not arise de novo. I am a student of phenomenology and have learned from readings, researching, attending workshops, giving workshops, teaching classes, and living through the world in an existential way.

This particular part of the book will be a collection of thoughts and ideas that I have integrated for myself in this process. They will not be in any particular order, for "order," in the way the word is used, implies normative commitments to the priority of ideas.

I lay no claim to the originality of the ideas presented in this book. They have become such a part of my perspective, I no longer know their origin in every instance. However, I hope that readers will use the bibliography at the end of the book to further explore this subject matter. Another caveat is that many of these beginning introductory remarks are written elsewhere in this book when the context is appropriate for expansion. These remarks occur to me as thoughts I wish to share with you. I sometimes think that such an effort as this is rather audacious and indeed it may be, so I live with that. However, it is balanced with what I see as an expressed need by students and colleagues. Because I offer a class on research from a phenomenological perspective, the assumption is that I must be an authority. Hardly so—I am, as I said, a student of phenomenology and teaching enables me to explore with others, being and experiences and all the meaning therein.

I suggest readings here and elsewhere to accompany your reading of this book. During this introduction, I would suggest reading Chapters 1 through 5 in *Nursing Research: A Qualitative Perspective* (1993) by Carolyn Oiler Boyd and myself. (Please believe this is not an advertisement!) Although you can continue reading the present book without referring to *Nursing Research*, the first five chapters of that book can provide background information if this content area is entirely new to you. Although the present work is not a companion volume, per se, but a going on of *Nursing Research,* I do not wish to repeat what has already been published. Of particular interest in the earlier book is Boyd's chapter on phenomenology and a phenomenological study by Sarah Lauterbach in Chapter 5. At the end of the present text, another phenomenological study, this one by Lucy Warren, is presented as an example.

The text by Max van Manen (1990) will be cited throughout this work as well. So depending on your familiarity with this subject matter, you might want to read that text. Some readers may be well acquainted with this perspective and with the many works and writings by our distinguished colleagues and scholars. Others may be just beginning a thesis, a dissertation, or a research project using this approach for the first time. Whichever it is, however, one book to refer to for definition or clarification will not be enough. You must read and become immersed in this subject or philosophy to "hear" how others speak about it.

What truly reflects the phenomenological approach? I will take the liberty of presenting what phenomenology means to me within this chapter. I have no books around me; I want this to truly reflect my interpretation of what I have understood in reading and praxis thus far. No dogma is implied, merely an interpretation. Some people think that the results of phenomenology should be raised to a level of abstraction, philosophical or otherwise. I do not share this belief, as I think it should "feel" like coming home to oneself or knowing the home of another in everyday life. I attempt to understand myself and I attempt to understand you, and I search for the meanings of what is presented or concealed in all of this.

SOME THOUGHTS ABOUT AN EXTRAORDINARY QUESTION

Phenomenology is a philosophy. As a philosophy, it seems mainly to be interested in a "phenomenal" question "What is the meaning of being human?" I suggest to students that they focus on this question until they have truly entered that dimension of thinking, "What does it mean to be a human being?" That they wonder and ponder over this extraordinary question.

Pedantic transgressions can take place in answering the preceding question because all philosophies are ultimately about meaning in some way. Still, there is value in persistent questioning. Even the followers of the often contrasted analytic philosophy say they are about meaning although their approach is quite different. The analytic philosophical school, so to speak, believes that true understanding takes place by understanding parts or concepts. How much life is there to that process? Little. While phenomenolgy is interested in parts vis-à-vis experiences, the interest in parts has a greater aim: to understand a particular meaning in pursuit of understanding what it means to be human. And phenomenologists do this best when they stay close to the language and ways of being that they are attempting to understand. In this way, the more "concrete" emerges in contrast to the abstract. Good phenomenology is within the human experience—concrete, ordinary, everyday human experience.

Anticipating a question regarding the place of abstraction here, my response is: Do not humans think in the abstract? For some people, thinking, talking, and working with abstract ideas is common. Abstraction is a way of being in the world, the meaning of which becomes a phenomenological question.

All known ways of being in the world can be described and interpreted from the phenomenological philosophical perspective (some might add hermeneutical to include interpretation). Phenomenology, however, should not be an academic exercise: I believe, as do others, that we have chosen phenomenology so that we can do better as humans who are "being" in this world.

Understanding the meaning of something "human" can stand on its own merits. As members of the caring professions, we often have specific goals and aims: "Above all, do no harm" could be one. So, through increased understanding of the meaning of situation, we become more capable of empathy and can present alternative ways of being for people to consider in living through experience.

One of my students challenged me quite correctly on two points from an article I wrote in 1982: (1)"There is no attempt to change them," and (2) "People are self-determining" (Munhall, 1982). To explain the first quote, and within context, I responded that I have no intention of changing people. The reason is found in the second quote—these ideas go hand in hand. Human beings deserve all the "knowing" we can provide for them. When we seek meaning and present such meaning as possibilities of being, we offer to individuals consolation that others share their perception. We might also present the possibility of alternative ways of perceiving. These two avenues of perception are not mutually exclusive and the latter usually follows the former. The irony here is that this kind of discussion diverts us from the task at hand. We get bogged down in academic, abstract discussions that have little to do with the person presenting before us.

On the other hand, phenomenological description and interpretations are commonly, and popularly, offered to people in self-help books. Trying to find a way out of their sometime chaotic world, people look to these books to help them make decisions. In such books, there is an invitation to consider a perception or many perceptions of a situated context and then to make an individual decision. If readers want to change a behavior or a way of thinking, it is, at least superficially, their decision. We, in the various caring professions, should be able to support and assist people in reaching their goals. If people want to change, we can help them. It is through the study of what it is "like" that we will best be able to assist them.

A popular book that offers phenomenological descriptions and interpretations is *It's Not What You're Eating, It's What's Eating You*, by Janet Greenson (1990, 1993). The Greenson book is a wonderful example of finding out the *meaning* of eating for some people. It calls to mind the futility of reducing calories or designing diets without exploring the emotional needs that eating may fulfill for individuals. The same may be said for the so-called eating disorders. The eating or not eating is a manifestation of something that needs to be understood. The meaning of that "thing" or "need" is showing itself in that way. That meaning influences behavior is critical to understand.

Although it is almost axiomatic to hear "all behavior has meaning," the majority of researchers and health care providers still *focus on the behavior*. Phenomenology, however, directs our attention to *meaning*. Understanding meaning has far greater value than focusing on the behavior.

If we understand the meaning of a behavior or an experience, we are certainly on surer footing for doing whatever might be more useful. Instead of placing patients, clients, or individuals on diets, we might write a book, such as the one mentioned, suggest counseling unrelated to dieting, suggest a support group *related to the meaning* rather than say, the *eating,* and offer other alternatives related to meaning.

This is why, I believe, the human sciences are now looking to the philosophy of phenomenology to guide their research endeavors. Some of us find this kind of inquiry more in synchrony with our own interpretation of what it means to be human. Although in some situations we do not have the time nor is it appropriate to search for meaning, the larger picture reemerges, so to speak, after the emergency has passed. That is why reflection as part of phenomenology is critical. For I would not ask a person who is on a diet to reflect on its meaning, lest I risk changing the experience for him or her. Since I have read somewhere that as much as 95 percent of diets fail, and I assume as well that dieting has other meanings, if I wish to understand the meaning of dieting, I would talk with people who have dieted and found that it was not a satisfactory solution.

At the same time, other colleagues are doing research on a term called "obesity" or another term called "eating disorders," and they are using different perspectives to understand the phenomenon, such as casual models or correlational and experimental studies. In the best of all possible worlds, these studies would form a whole. Yet instead of working together, researchers using these perspectives are often isolated from one another and, worse, are competitive.

Phenomenology is not a research "method." It is often defined as the study of lived experience. How a person studies that lived experience depends more on philosophical assumptions than on methods. However, in the history of our development, some psychologists did indeed embrace phenomenology and perhaps developed methods to gain acceptance by the scientific community. Although the language, linearity, and structural modes of these methods are present, many individuals find the outcomes unimpressive. As I have previously said elsewhere in this book, this approach was part of the scientific community, or situated context, and researchers could not wander far from the scientific method of logical positivism. To learn about the experience of being human, a person went to the theater, read fiction or biographies, or even watched television.

Without becoming too distracted by the word "method," I want to point out a serious danger in using it in a phenomenological study. The method of a study is usually developed before the study begins. If you are planning to study lived experience and are naive (which you are supposed to be) about the experience, you will not know beforehand, the steps, language, sample, setting, or analysis of the data needed. How you come to understand an experience will be guided by what individuals tell you about the experience. They talk, you listen. In addition, once you have decided to study an experience, you become open to its appearance everywhere, and it is always appearing. You begin to see and hear it in films, photographs, other people's conversations, newspapers, and so on. It becomes difficult to know prospectively what will make itself known. Retrospectively, however, a researcher can say how he or she came to understand an experience. Figure 2.1 is not a method, but provides a map of different places a researcher might consider in coming to know meaning.

If phenomenology has been defined as the study of lived experience, what about the meaning component? For example, with empirical phenomenology or descriptive phenomenology, a researcher may go through all there is to know and understand about an experience. The process has an epistemological quality of obtaining knowledge about something. The *meaning part*—what does it mean to be human—is instead an *ontological question.* This latter emphasis of phenomenology usually has a hermeneutical phase. Not only does a researcher describe experience but he or she attempts to interpret the meaning of that experience. I offer students the following guidelines:

- I don't believe phenomenology, as the study of lived experience, can be obtained by interpreting six to ten transcribed interviews.
- Nor do I place much faith in the outline I give to students to follow although it may often be helpful, especially in the beginning. So I allow this *pro*spective document to be written because the students seem more secure (see Appendix B). I don't object to their feeling insecure, but I don't wish to frustrate students with a philosophy that they can speak but find difficult to practice because of their prior socialization.

- Van Manen's (1991) steps are also useful and do not differ much
  from the items in Figure 2.1. The shape of the diagram as it appears in this book, however, demonstrates the concentricity of
  concurrent activities and sources of data.

Since this chapter is designed to simplify some ideas, let's return
to lived experience and the meaning of being human. An enigma, a
big riddle—call it what you will—we still have a path toward this
aim. (I do not like to say a means toward an end since it does not

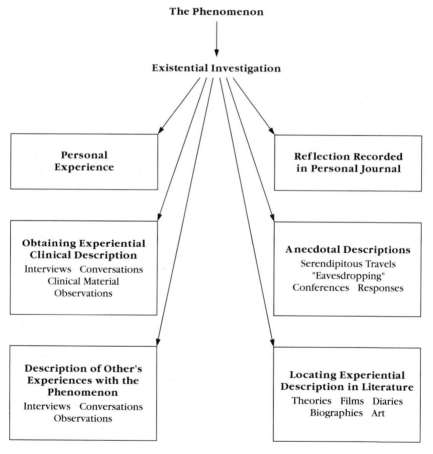

Figure 2.1.   The Phenomenon: Existential Investigation.

ring humanistic.) So if our aim as researchers doing phenomenoloy in a descriptive study guided by the phenomenological perspective is to contribute to the understanding of what it means to be human, we do this by studying the experience that humans have. We cannot study the meaning of being human in a serious way unless we study what humans do, how they interpret their experiences, and what meaning they attach to the experience. Researchers often make incorrect assumptions about meaning on this basis: They say the person may have chosen the experience. Individuals make similar decisions for very different reasons and experience the meaning differently as well.

In this regard, researchers need to be open to varying perceptions of the same phenomenon or experience when collecting material and listening to individuals. Individuals have different backgrounds and situated contexts that will influence their perceptions. The important thing about perception in a phenomenological study is to respect each individual's interpretation of an event as his or her own reality or truth.

Another word people hear when learning about phenomenology is "consciousness." It has been said that consciousness is the only access individuals have to the world. However, while we may be conscious of some "thing," our unconscious is always at work. This realization needs to be part of our research in that we periodically check ourselves as to how we are listening and interpreting. Through whose lens? Our own defense mechanisms, which are largely unconscious, can prevent us from seeing reality from another perspective (see discussions on readiness in Chapter 5, and unknowing in Chapter 4).

The outcome of studies from the perspective of consciousness is usually "raised" consciousness. We become more aware, more conscious, we understand things that were hidden to us. Perhaps responses such as, "I never thought about it that way before," "It never dawned on me till I read your study," and the like are examples of raised consciousness.

Intersubjectively, another concept is simply what happens whenever two people engage in interaction or one person hears another's interpretation of experience. In our studies, when we listen, truly to be present, we attempt to set aside our subjective assumptions or presuppositions. However, the dialogue is essential, and the intersubjective meeting space, where one person listens and the other person tells his or her story is the heart of the study (see Chapter 4 for further discussion of intersubjectivity).

Embodiment is yet another concept of importance. We are in the world through our bodies. The individuals we converse with are in their bodies all revealing and concealing at once. We speak of body language. We make many assumptions about the other based on appearance. To know another, we must once again hold these assumptions in abeyance.

Because of our orientation to "method," we chose "methods" for doing phenomenology that were created by phenomenologically oriented psychologists. Their mode of thinking has led to various methods that rely primarily on procedures with systematic steps that arrive at a "structure" of the experience. Basically, then, the methods reported as used in health care journals are those that have evolved from empirical-phenomenological psychology. These methods include those developed by van Kaam, Colazzi, and Georgi.

- As demonstrated by van Manen (1990), existential phenomenology widens the lens of understanding with the inclusion of literature, art, myths, film, poetry, and journals.

- Thus far in human science research, a researcher's phenomenological perspective can be identified by the choice of one of these orientations: Van Kaam, Georgi, Colozzi, or van Manen. Many nurse researchers have elaborated on these methods as well, including Benner (1993), Diekelmann (1985), Oiler (1993), Ray (1985), and Parse (1987).

- Within this text, I embrace both the existential and the hermeneutical approaches in different ways than investigators in the field of psychology have developed them. In the discipline of psychology, as it relates to phenomenology, researchers have attempted to focus on "essential meaning-constituents" (van Kaam), "meaning units" (Georgi), or "themes and scenes" (Fisher). The seemingly mechanistic language is accompanied by a specific method with specific steps. It is reminiscent of "*the* scientific method."

However, the essential question is the extent to which any method helps us to understand what it means to be human. Understanding the meaning of being human is the paramount aim of this research perspective. In this regard, the ideas presented here are all the result of three kinds of dialogue:

1. *Internal Dialogue.* This refers to myself thinking and responding to all that has gone before me and whatever continues to present itself.
2. *External Dialogue.* Here many types of dialogues have taken place. One type of dialogue has been with students whose work and questions are included in this text. Another dialogue has been with persons who have helped me understand human experience, whether they were research participants, teachers, patients, someone I do not know well, yet may come to know better.
3. *The Eternal Dialogue.* This seems never to stop. I may not even be conscious of it, but it surfaces when it is supposed to and I am open to it with consciousness. Lyrics of songs talk to me of life. The books that surround me tell me stories of what it means to be human. Emotions, displayed and felt by others and myself, show meaning. The construction of reality in films and novels tells me about the conflicts, fantasies, and dreams of humans. Myths are sometimes like that. Anecdotes, these short stores I hear, reflect what humans value. And I could go on. What I would like to say here is that my being in the work in a phenomenological way does seem eternal. I don't try to escape it, and in fact I surrender to it in a serendipitous manner.

However, a word to the wise. "Readiness" is spoken about in this text. Phenomenology is not for everyone, or individuals may not be ready for phenomenology. I'm reminded of this in classes. Though there is laughter, there are also tears and pain. As human beings, we need to respect how others "are" in this world. If a person chooses a research method from a perspective that inherently espouses distance, we need to respect that purpose both in terms of the method and the researcher. My aim here is not to convert all researchers to phenomenology nor to help people get closer to finding meaning. Remember, finding meaning is a personal choice.

We are not acting as therapists in the researcher's role. We have dialogue and conversation with the aim of increasing understanding. If in the process of this conversation we come upon strong defense mechanisms, that is part of our understanding of the experience. That is part of the description, *not something in the moment that needs to be changed.* Researching from a phenomenological perspective does not include "breaking down" defenses or suggesting to people other ways of "being."

Social or therapeutic communication or conversation may include presenting an alternative perspective for the other to consider, but in a dialogue for research guided by *phenomenology,* we listen, prompt the person to continue, so that the conversation from this perspective is really one of a storyteller with a curious listener who asks "and?" or "could you give me an example?"

I sometimes wonder what to do with the word "method." Van Manen (1990) says that writing is the method: "Language is a central concern in phenomenological research because responsive-reflective writing is the very activity of doing phenomenology" (p. 132).

In addition, van Manen cautions us about the tendency toward abstractions, yet this is often a criterion or step written as part of the "methods" available to us. In this book I hope to be concrete. Though often I wander into Heidegger's language, I still hope to be concrete and real. A personal anecdote: When I first started writing articles, I tried my best to be abstract, to be intellectual, and to do what was valued by many journals (i.e., be "scientific"). Today, I want to be more imaginative, concrete, in the real world. I don't want to set up barriers with language. I wish to write to be understood, not necessarily to be agreed with, but to be understood.

Practically every book on the nonfiction best seller list in the self-help category could have been written by a nurse or health care professional. They are either examples of studies that could be considered phenomenological or include phenomenological material. They are purposely close to experience and written in plain talk.

We thus need to consider our audiences. Perhaps what you are studying, searching for an understanding of, belongs to the people and not to the academics. Perhaps as we write, we need to consider, for example, families in need of our descriptions and interpretations. Perhaps we need to write to the people.

There is a paradox here in that clearly written plain talk is not viewed as true scholarly writing. It is interesting to note that when an academic writes a book, it tends to be reviewed as remote or esoteric, whereas a book written by a journalist on the same topic soars to the best seller list. Most of the time, I think the latter owes its success to using plain talk, getting close to the reader, being concrete, and not creating a feeling of inadequacy by distancing the reader from the material. Engaging a reader is very important to the phenomenological writer. "Engaging" talk avoids raising language to intellectual abstractions and reconstructing experience to convoluted prose.

Time to get off the dock. I have attempted, in this chapter, to liberate myself from restraints to creativity. Once again I will go to the airport, this time to pick up Chuck and Ray whose plane is late—interesting, the idea of "airplanes," of "flying back and forth." Am I not doing the same? Over the development of this book, the simple, ordinary event of the airport trip assumed much greater significance. I was able to see it in contexts other than that proscribed by "simple" or "ordinary." Always look for the extraordinary in the ordinary. "Something" only becomes ordinary because it occurs so often. Those occurrences that happen so frequently are the fabric of being human. And it is in this fabric that we are able to question being in a phenomenological way.

3

What's It All About, Alfie?
The Phenomenological Question

In this chapter, we explore the "living" of the phenomenological question. The psychodynamic aspect of a study from the phenomenological perspective includes the idea that meaning is often concealed in behavior. Grasping this complex essence of experience is the path to meaning. To know the meaning of an experience is the way to understand the meaning of being human.

"Being here," "being there," and "being-in-the-world" are discussed in relation to becoming phenomenologically oriented and living that out in a meaningful way. We do not study the meaning of being as an intellectual exercise. We study the meaning of being so that we become more human and life in an everyday world becomes more meaningful.

"What's it all about, Alfie?" is to ask, What is life in terms of being in this world? If meaning is often concealed in behavior, it becomes an important concept to understand in our human interconnectedness.

*T*he first question of any phenomenological encounter or study is the question of being, so the understandings we seek through phenomenology are essentially those of being. We ask questions that have to do with a particular experience of our being in the world.

Heidegger (1927) gives us some thoughtful and insightful accounts of the nature of our being. These ideas are part of all phenomenological thinking in that they belong to a basic ontology of the meaning of being. Much of the literature from the phenomenological perspective in the human sciences state openly that a study is one of a particular experience. If the student of the experience probes further, he or she will look for the meaning of the experience and perhaps capture an understanding of the essential question—the meaning of being human. Preceding any lived experience is this fundamental question about the meaning of being: "Being is always the being of an entity" (p. 29).

So it is in this being of an entity that we have certain areas of subject matter to study. Because our everyday language is not always consistent with phenomenological language, we often transpose the language of the scientific method to phenomenological inquiry. Science is one way to study being or the being of an entity, but it has limitations if we wish to understand the larger questions of being in existence. We then come upon the existential, the concreteness of everyday existence, the being "there," the "dailiness," our consciousness and awareness.

I recall a line in a play where one of the characters asks another why she married her husband. The reply was, "Because he was there." The reason for climbing a mountain is often also, "It was there." Heidegger refers to person as "Dasein," meaning a person's being "there" as a mode for attempting to understand being.

We are always somewhere; therefore, we are always being there. This concept is intrinsic to the idea of studying lived experience, and it is in experience that we name "being there." This is the world in which we are or in which we may be or find ourselves. It is this world that we in the human sciences want, perhaps are compelled, to understand. Also it is not the objects that interest us as much as the experiences of human existence and how we *are* with objects— we focus on our relatedness, say to technology, to science, with one another, embodied in experiences.

Why does a human science pursue such questions? Because we acknowledge this relatedness to one another, or experience of being, involving our human concern and a search for meaning. Dasein, it has been noted, is ontologically related to the entities by an attitude of care. Research thus becomes a caring act, or an act of caring to know more about what it means "to be" in the world. We search to solve the mysteries, not for control but for understanding the unmeasurable or the concealed. The task is always pursuing the question of the meaning of being. We acknowledge temporality as a beacon in this task: Time is a horizon for all understanding of being. Looking to the human world entities, we then become embedded in existential (real-life) experiences as they unfold in their dailiness. Time for us, even when asleep, in dreams, is an experience of mind, thoughts, values, feelings, memories, actions, wishes, regrets, and emotions. We attempt to understand "being" in humans' consciousness as they exist in this world within the dimension of temporality.

While it has been said that phenomenology was a reaction to logical positivism, the temporality of the situated context at that point of history is acknowledged. Today, we could propose that phenomenology is an essential philosophy or perspective from which we guard ourselves against the dehumanization of technology, vacant morality, and arbitrary norms. Sachs in his book asks, "Is there anybody home?" In a hospital, his being is now connected from one piece of technology to another, so that he wonders if a human being is present anywhere. Occasionally, someone's voice comes through the wall of a hospital in response to a patient's intercom switch. The voice says, "Yes?" And the patient responds to empty air and a receiver. This human situation begs for study. What is the meaning of this? This scenario, repeated in many ways, calls for attentive awareness to these everyday details, and the trivial observation of being there can become "How could this be?"

Living the phenomenological question is living the question of "what is being?" When we choose to research from a phenomenological perspective, the "being" means the being of entities. These entities themselves are researched to help us understand the meaning of being. Being is itself an entity, capable of being known through other entities.

While phenomenology is the study of lived experience, we need to understand that the study of a lived experience is always the study of being. We return to the patient in his bed wondering if anyone is home. We have the question of an experience as "being" through existing itself. So attentiveness to this state of everydayness, to this being of entity, guides us in the search for the meaning of being.

Often, I have found students struggling with what lived experience they want to study even though they know they wish to study some "thing" from a phenomenological perspective. That thing, if brought to awareness, should be prompted by a genuine quest to first and foremost understand what it means to be human. When choosing a specific entity or existential experience, we come closer to that, and indeed the living of the experience itself may be what we remain focused on in this search for understanding. What I have found extraordinary though is an experience where "the thing itself is deeply veiled" (Heidegger, p. 49).

When we start seeking the meaning and interpretation of some named experience, we may come upon a hidden phenomenon. We must stay open to the appearance of "things," of what shows itself and what is brought forth. The step commonly referred to as "bracketing" allows for both the manifest and nonmanifest to be described and interpreted as they appear or do not appear.

Van Manen (1990) tells us that the ultimate aim of phenomenological research is: "the fulfillment of our human nature: to become more fully who we are" (p. 12).

This becomes a struggle for human scientists as they try to raise awareness and consciousness to the depersonalization and estrangements acknowledged within the pressures and influences of science, technology, economics, and politics.

Just what does all this mean? Phenomenology, a methodological concept, is the study of being, and being exists in situations that may be called entities. They exist in time or history; they occur within a specific context.

Often, we refer to these situations as lived experiences. Through studying these lived experiences of other human beings, we may come to understand what it means to be human. If we understand such meaning, our consciousness is expanded and the possibility of becoming more fully human presents itself. And so, we are back to a familiar idea that van Manen (1990) expressed this way:

> In this sense human science research is itself a kind of Buldung on paideia; it is the curriculum of being and becoming. (p. 7)

This perspective is grounded in many assumptions about being, some of which were discussed in Chapter 1, and now will be linked in a way that I believe needs to be embedded and simultaneously questioned as we are about to embark on a study of some phenomenon.

As we attempt our search for meaning, these assumptions must be like perception that the self knows in a way that has penetrated what I think of as the *cognitive barrier*. Consider the following ideas:

- Perception centers meaning.
- Perception, cognition (what we think we know), and language (in all forms) are forms of access to meaning.
- The evolving of your question is founded in the life-world, that is, where you are in daily experience and action. It is before you, and yet you are in it as well.
- The question or your interests are situated in context. The context is all, it is the time, the space, the body, the human relation.
- The context changes with different times, space, bodies, and relationships.
- Your search finds some meaning in "some" thing but not all things because they are different and changing depending on the context.
- To ask a question from this perspective is to be conscious of something and to turn your attention to this something, and this turning is an intentional act.
- In evolving a quest for such understanding, you need to lighten up on the need for order, certainty, answers from others guiding your research, and books such as this one, and let things come as they appear. This is reflective of being-in-the-world and open to what appears.
- A phenomenological attitude needs to be tended to. Having been rewarded for knowing things, we are asked to "unknow" things and perhaps liberate ourselves from the very knowledge that can and often does depersonalize and dehumanize experience.
- Tending to a phenomenological attitude is like floating in water: Let yourself float, let the adviser float, let there be silence, peace, and contemplation.
- Though we all know we cannot "live" without steps in a research project, let us not deliberate in endless dialogues, monologues, or trivial disagreements on the possibility of bracketing, hammering out themes, and applying techniques to data.

- The phenomenological attitude, so to speak, is to listen, to hear, to see the phenomenon wherever it appears, to be ever open for an appearance, and to be as unfettered as possible with preconceptions.
- To study meaning this way is to become the question you are asking.

What the study of meaning is not:

- It is not following steps.
- It is not slavishly following the steps of the scientific method nor using its language or criteria.
- It is not solely ten transcribed interviews.
- It does not restrict a phenomenon to a definition, categories, or constructs.
- It is not found in a definition.

THE PHENOMENOLOGICAL QUESTION

If the phenomenological question for the purpose of this text is the meaning of being human, then the question should always have that dimension within it.

Let us return to the student described in Chapter 2.

This student was working with homeless women (already a category). She was a nurse and said she was interested in studying the lived experience of homeless women as they experience nursing. She added that she wanted to understand how they perceive the nursing care they receive.

Because I think students need guidance, though not direction, I asked her: "Why not study what it means to live without a home, or a space in the world that is their own? What is the meaning of this experience, that we as a culture call "homelessness"? I asked her what she thought of doing her study from this perspective and to acknowledge her own interests. I added, "Perhaps nursing care will emerge as giving meaning to the experience of not having a home."

At this point, I hope you will reflect on your own experiences and just substitute different words, where needed, to describe your study. In this case, the student was fairly adamant, convinced, and committed to what she wanted to study.

The scenario represents a fairly common experience that I have lived through many times. I always present my perception, but in the end I let students have freedom. I do this purposefully because, first, I respect these students, and second, I am open and am trying to demonstrate the phenomenological attitude. The student is off pursuing ten (a magic number from somewhere) interviews with women without homes, asking them about their nursing care. When presenting her work the other night, she lamented: "It's hard to keep the subjects focused on the question. They just want to talk about being homeless."

I admired her tenacity; she still would not change her original question and I was still open to the idea that the study might help us understand the meaning of some human experience. It is often the case that what we began with, our "beginningness," leads where we can find deeper meanings.

Heidegger (1927) said:

In spite of the fact that "appearing" is never showing-itself in the sense of "phenomenon," appearing is possible only by reason of a showing-itself of something. (p. 53)

He states further:

This is what one is talking about when one speaks of the symptoms of a disease. Here one has in mind certain occurrences in the body which show themselves and which, in showing themselves "indicate" something which does not show itself. (p. 52)

Quite simply then, we might say, "Things are seldom what they seem to be." Strictly interpreted, however, phenomenology concerns itself with appearance, yet it is always alert to covered-up-ness as the counterconcept to phenomenon. A critical consideration for the human scientist is the extent to which he or she does not include what is concealed, intuited to be concealed, or interpreted to be concealed in the interpretation of material gathered in a study. This will be discussed further.

Back though to formulating the phenomenological question, whose aim, as suggested earlier, is the question of being. Calling upon Heidegger's Dasein, the being of Dasein has an existential meaning of care.

Van Manen (1990) says: "Then research is a caring act: we want to know that which is most essential to being" (p. 5).

Thus, we approach formulating the research question from the phenomenological perspective: *What is it about being-in-the-world that matters deeply to us?* To be involved in research—to experience doing research—a person ideally should come upon a human experience that he or she profoundly desires to understand. To hear researchers say, "I don't know what lived experience to study," or "Would you suggest a lived experience?" is to miss the passion of research and take on academic exercising.

Doing phenomenological research can be transformative; I would dare say it should be. So what you choose to study should be close to your heart or soul and thus centered in human "being."

We want to become more fully human, more conscious, in a place and time where beings are more and more depersonalized and estranged. Researchers, from this perspective, are like fish swimming upstream. Heidegger places great emphasis on this:

> *The ontology of Dasein may then be understood as a symbol of an anguished struggle for individuality and grounded authenticity in a world where one is in perceptual danger of absorption in the pressures and influences of the social milieu. (Atwood & Stolorow, 1989, p. 23)*

So it helps to have passion and a heartfelt, soulful interest in a human experience before embarking on a study of it. I would say it is essential.

In concrete terms, the question will ask the "whatness" of being in the experience: "What is it like to _____?"

Dialogue follows in an attempt to grasp the intensity, the meaning, and the essence of experiencing being. It is important to keep centered on the original question of being-in-the-experience.

Name the experience and place cards about your own life-world to remind you what it is that you are attending to. We may say that such research requires attentiveness, yet we can be led astray. Attentiveness and intentionality can be transformed to absorption. We become absorbed in the quest for understanding what it means to experience some "thing."

We begin to live the phenomenological question. We are attentive to its appearance whenever or wherever it appears! This is where some of the more structured ways of doing phenomenology may seem fundamentally, historically odd. Structural definitions and categories or even lists of themes do not reflect how people live through experiences. They do in fact depersonalize us or dehumanize us by often demonstrating what we are not. What if our experience does not fit the definition? So we research and write to include many possibilities of being in the experience. We must also give up the idea that everyone who reads our writing will grasp its every aspect with recognition and "Oh, yes, that's how it is."

Some people who have talked to us or have had the experience may respond to our research and writing by saying, "Oh, yes, *some* of that happened to me." And still yet, if it wasn't that way for them, we need to find out what it was like for them.

When a study of a real experience is truly a contribution and is reported verbally, people in the audience, whether they had the experience or not, are moved by the description, are affected by the words describing the experience, and "become" with the study. I have been moved to tears and laughter with students, often a mixture, when phenomenological material is read or presented. Ironically, placing it in the academic format seems to remove the lifeblood. But perhaps that is part of our struggle to gain academic acceptance for research of being-in-the-world that is not observational, intellectual, abstract, and removed from human experience.

GRASPING THE ESSENCE OF EXPERIENCE

In our effort to understand what it means to grasp the essence of the experience, it seems fitting to return to the fundamental underlying question of the meaning of being. In Heidegger's (1927) *Being and Time,* we read:

*In so far as Being constitutes what it is asked about and being
means the Being of entities then entities themselves turn out to be
what is interrogated. (p. 26)*

And, as quoted earlier: "Being is always the being of an entity" (p.
29).

Our access to this knowing is through our consciousness and
awareness. It is within us, our bodies, where we are; our being is not
split either mind-body, inner-outer, subjective-objective. Our being-
body is in time-place and in relation to other being-bodies.

As was mentioned in the previous chapter, our access to knowing
through our perception and unconsciousness must always be informed by the idea that the "thing itself" may be deeply veiled. However, we have come up with a question and now are faced with the
quest to understand what we are asking and what about this experience will assist us in understanding being.

This is a task of no small consequence requiring from curious
investigators a soulfulness and mindfulness to be ever attentive to
being-in-the-world in a certain manner. Dailiness, the taken for
granted, and the "not seen" call for our perception and awareness.
What has remained silent, we begin to hear.

*To have a science of phenomena means to grasp its object in such a
way that everything about them which is up for discussion must be
treated by exhibiting it directly and demonstrating it directly.
(Heidegger, 1927, p. 59)*

We come across the word "hermeneutics" when we take the preceding description of a phenomenon and attempt an interpretive
characterization of existence in the world. So through this embrace,
we participate and the world comes into existence. We then in a hermeneutic way try to make sense of it.

Let us imagine what we are truly studying through looking at experience as participation in the world. Grasping the experience of
existence might include these ideas:

• The grasp is human.
• The grasp is to understand being.

- To understand being, we see "being" in participation.
- We decide to participate in an activity of being that is called phenomenology.
- We can perhaps get glimpses of the meaning of being through participation in the world.
- Human participation is in experience.
- We get closer to understanding if we increase our awareness of experience.
- We get closer to understanding through interpretation of the meaning of beings in their participation.
- The best way to accomplish this is to remain open to all notions of the experience as they appear.
- Openness requires suspending what we think we know—our presuppositions, assumptions, and theories.
- We start by asking, "What is it like?"

This chapter includes several suggestions that are relevant to both theory and practice and will be referred to as we progress. Few situations can be more frustrating for students than not knowing where to start and where to go and, if course, how to do it. What follows is applicable for research, practice, and teaching. Once an individual lets phenomenology serve as a way of being-in-the-world, it is difficult (at least it has been for me) to step out of it.

So I would like to posit to the novice: Be patient; for the most part, you were not brought up with this worldview as a way of being. After ten years, I have learned from colleagues, students, readings, and what appears that my choice to participate in this worldview is a lifelong being. It is not a religion, though some have suggested that it is somewhat Zen. Phenomenology is a philosophy, or a research approach. Put simply, all these categories and words mean I have chosen to look for the meaning of being here, in this time, place, and in relations with others. I have chosen this focus so I can find meaning for myself and assist patients and students who may also choose to journey through time this way. It is a way of being that acknowledges the primacy of being. It takes very seriously the question, "Is anyone home?"

At this point in your search for meaning, assume you have decided to study a lived experience. As part of this effort, the following resources will be helpful:

1. For a phenomenological perspective, *Being and Time* (Heidegger, 1927) or a related text on this work.
2. *Researching Lived Experience* (van Manen, 1984).
3. Published studies using this approach (i.e., a Heideggerian or van Manen approach).
4. Articles listed as sources within the preceding works.
5. As previously suggested, Chapters 1-5 in *Nursing Research: A Qualitative Perspective* (Munhall & Oiler-Boyd, 1993).

Before proceeding, ask yourself if you have more questions now and if you feel somewhat confused. Whether you are a novice or an expert, this uncertainty is all to the good. Remember Morgan's (1983) axiom:

Assumptions make messes researchable, often as the cost of great oversimplification, and in a way that is highly problematic. (Morgan, p. 377)

Several procedures are appropriate in your next phase (not to imply a linear process). The phases are always in process as you add to, reflect on, change, and think intensely about your study. Revisiting and enriching the suggested phases is part of the daily livingness of your inquiry. Try the following:

• Write out fully your personal experience with the phenomenon; you should reveal your personal self as being in the study to the extent that you are comfortable. Why this experience, for what purpose?
• Suspend your beliefs—sometimes called "bracketing." I have heard researchers who have presented studies from a phenomenological perspective state, "Bracketing is not possible so it was rejected." "Unknowing" may be a better word than bracketing. You need to stand before an experience with an

attitude of unknowing, even and especially if you have lived that experience yourself. Different possibilities need the opportunity to emerge. Also, and I will repeat this, your own lived experience description is not a phenomenological description, it is material from which to work. It is essential to approach your own knowing and living of an experience as illustrated in Chapter 4, "Unknowing."

- Reflect on the common everyday usage of the word or phrases socially embedded in the context from which you are positioned. What is the origin of the word and what are some phrases that are in common usage about this phenomenon? The culture in which you are situated has already assigned some meaning to what you are about to study, whether it be mythical, normative, or metaphorical.

- Be-in-the-world with your experience. This being is a knowing conscious, inquisitive being. Material is before you, and you begin to see, hear, and converse about it. This is the grasping of the experience; suggested avenues are illustrated in Figure 2.1.

- The four existential life-worlds (see Figure 3.1) are interwoven throughout your study always highlighting your situated context. Though circled in the figure for accentuation, the four life-worlds are but *one, the life-world* you are in. Articulating the particulars of that life-world can contribute to your understanding of the phenomenon. Van Manen (1990) states: "Spatiality, corporality, temporality, and relationality are productive categories for the process of phenomenological question posing, reflecting, and writing" (p. 102).

In the translation of these concepts, we are acknowledging the experience of the space we are in (where are we), the time we are in, our past, present, and future, the body that enables us to be in the world, and where and when we are interpersonally connected. It is critical to acknowledge the subjective nature of these life-worlds and that the perceptions of any of them will differ among people who are even very close to us. For example, their past is different and therefore influences their perception of the present. Their gender may be different, as well as their cultural space. To know this is to understand

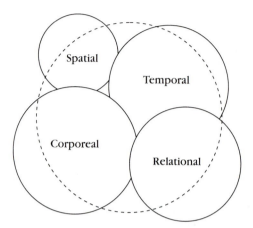

Figure 3.1. The Life Worlds.

that we are living in the moment, our present, which also contains someone's future and someone's past. Linear time has little to do with this notion. Imagine a swimming pool with children ages three to five years, adults in mid-life, and older adults, who are retired. Perception of time, space, body, and relationships are pungently and profoundly different for these groups, all at once in one moment that we call "the present." Immediately, it is gone; it becomes the past that we can reflect on and what was the future now is the present.

Though I might say this again, studying an individual's experience in the present changes it and thus does not allow us to understand it in an authentic manner. Again, if we were to ask any of the people in the swimming pool what it felt like to be there, we would have interrupted and changed the experience. In my work on anger (Munhall, 1993b), I explained that if I were to ask individuals, "What is it like to be angry?" when they were experiencing the anger, the stopping to reflect would change their experience. Some people think asking questions while "it is" (the experience) actually going on, enables them to grasp the true essence. However, in doing that, we are saying, "Stop what is going on, stop experiencing the experience, and instead talk about what this anger means to you, feels to you. What's it like?" And thus the experience is changed, stopped. The irony of this approach is that in some situations this might make sense, but it does not always in a research study from a phenomenological perspective. In the extreme, if an angry person were about to hurt him- or herself, or someone else, we would interrupt the outburst—we would be present during the experience. But in our research as part of the coming to know about the experience, we often seek people who have *had* the experience and are able to talk about it.

Perhaps the experience you wish to study is a broader one that is part of an individual's life-world. The contrast here may be one of an episode or a life circumstance.

In a study I am now doing on finding meaning in midlife for women, I sense, as the study unfolds, that for some women the lived experience is not a reflecting back on something that is over but a telling of a story that is a life circumstance. "What is it like to be a parent?" is also a circumstance that changes in the four existential life-worlds, yet in most instances, we can feel comfortable that an interview or conversation about such a circumstance will not change it in any way other than perhaps beneficially.

Of course, if talking about a circumstance has the potential of causing harm, then we ethically cannot pursue such study. There are such sensitive topics, and unless you are educated in this particular experience and know as a professional that talking will be therapeutic, inquiry is inappropriate (see Chapter 9 regarding ethical considerations).

This is where I find the life-world of being a psychotherapist and nurse helpful. Teachers or guidance counselors may have life-worlds that permit them to assess whether it is in the best interest of the individual to talk about an experience. Social workers, nurse practitioners, and clinical specialists also are able to make appropriate determinations.

Suppose, however, you want to study the experience of a circumstance in life such as menopause. Gail Sheehy's (1992) book is an excellent example of how to study an experience with benefits accruing. Though her book is not labeled a phenomenological study, in a casual sense it is one. It answers the question to a large extent "What is it like to experience menopause?"

Her interpretation though is purely her own, and as optimistic as it may be, it does not represent mutual interpretation, characteristic of a good phenomenological study. Nevertheless, we have much to learn from her, through the experience of the life-worlds of the women she spoke with. Her piece of writing about a lived experience, which is more like a lived circumstance, incorporates and reintegrates being in the world with:

- Thoughts.
- Consciousness.
- Values.
- Feelings.
- Emotions
- Actions.
- Purposes.

Sheehy (1992) uses language, arts, institutions, consultations, group meetings, and literature in addition to interviews. These are all paths to knowing. Some potential areas for exploration include:

- Personal experiences.
- Clinical descriptions—interviews, conversations, observations.
- Description of other's experiences with the phenomenon.
- Anecdotal descriptions—serendipitous narratives.
- Experiential description in literature, films, theories, biographies, and art.

It is through the living of the question that a meaning becomes possible. We need to live the question with all that presents itself in appearances and all that the appearances conceal. It is important, I believe, to go beyond interviews in phenomenological inquiry if we are to enrich the narrative of being here, being there, and being-in-the-world. But I get ahead of myself. If you have come upon a human experience that you care deeply about, then you are ready to question it in a phenomenological way. How we find answers is the subject of the next chapter.

4

They Came in Through the Backdoor Window

After the Question, Where to Go

By this being-in-time, you will have become aware of the repetition of thoughts presented here. They are repeated, however, in different contexts so that you can think about what is said from the front door, backdoor, and windows.

I once said that to a student who was encountering difficulty with where to start. There is no starting place, so to speak. There are many portals of entry and many places to go once the question is asked, or the phenomenon is named.

One frequent starting place, however, is the naming of the experience, which often leads to the phenomenological question. I say one way, because that naming of an experience may lead to another experience that holds your interest in a more meaningful way.

This chapter discusses bracketing and decentering as ways of "unknowing." It discusses ways that you can get out of your own way, become the "unknower" and look to others and other material as the "knowers." The chapter also considers intersubjectivity as part of coming to know another and your need to decenter to allow that to happen.

THE USES OF BRACKETING IN PHENOMENOLOGY

We have been socialized in research to develop a proposal before we do our research. Oftentimes, there might even be a stopgap at an early phase where the researcher must defend his or her proposal or submit it for human subjects' review.

The proposal frequently is longer than what follows. It is detailed and leaves little unplanned for. It takes on a life of its own and reflects a paradigm, a bound-up plan. What if along the way something occurs that was not planned for? Should the researcher follow up on it if it wasn't part of the original plan?

From a phenomenological perspective, that is what should occur. We are asking a question. The answers we receive provide direction; they show us how to proceed. Some "thing" appears to us; we become aware of something when we are a part of it. We become aware of something because, rather than its being revealed, we understand that there is a covered-up-ness.

To understand the precise and owned meaning a particular experience has for an individual, we need first to explore the meaning that experience has for us as we do the research. We consider whether we have had the experience personally or have a different reason for being interested in a specific experience. We need to understand what it is we are about before beginning a study of this nature.

So self is a critical part of a phenomenological approach to knowing. (That self is critical to all our endeavors seems quite obvious, yet there seems to be collusion among some scientists to prove that self is not a part of research—but that is not what this discussion is about.) In "bracketing," the researcher lays down for readers his or her self-assumptions about the experience, or the phenomenon: what he or she believes about the projected study or the basis for the study. The researcher answers these questions for readers: Why this study? Who are you in this study?

These assumptions are critical because they are untested, yet agreed upon, truths about reality. Nonetheless, they form a foundation for a study. There are some assumptions about phenomenology as well. For example, van Manen (1990) states what he believes phenomenology *is not* and what *it is*. That I agree with him (with one exception) does not equate to truth, however, but means that we share the same assumptions. They are as follows:

1. Phenomenology is not an empirical analytic science.
2. It is not mere speculative inquiry in the sense of unworldly reflection.
3. It is neither mere particularity nor sheer universality.
4. It does not problem solve (though this is a matter of interpretation; I believe it lays the groundwork for solving problems).

According to van Manen (1990), phenomenology is:

1. The study of lived experiences.
2. The explication of phenomena as they present themselves to consciousness.
3. The study of essences.
4. The description of the experiential meaning as we live it.
5. The human scientific study of phenomena.
6. The attentive practice of thoughtfulness.
7. A search for what it means to be human.
8. A poetizing activity.

Not only are you always questioning your assumptions about phenomenology but you are asked to bracket out your presuppositions about the phenomenon. Now this idea of bracketing is somewhat different.

This bracketing is supposedly the activity of explicating your assumptions and preunderstandings about the specific phenomenon or lived experience that you wish to study. Essentially, this activity should allow you to get out of your *own way* of perceiving something. You become attuned and conscious of your beliefs, and then wonder how it is for others. Knowing from the soul, that for others, it might be different and then being able to allow others their perceptions is the way to hearing in a phenomenological way. Your study has nothing to do with documenting your assumptions; it has to do with the meaning of being human, which will differ for individuals.

Peterson & Zderad (1976) stated:

In order to open the data of experience in using the phenomenological approach, one strives to eliminate "the a priori" (that which

exists in his mind prior to and independent of the experience) . . .
granted a person cannot be completely perspectiveless. Man is an
individual; he is a unique here and now person. So naturally, nec-
essarily, he has an "angular" view for he experiences reality from
the angle of his own particular "here" and his own particular
"now." However, by recognizing and considering the particular per-
spective from which he is experiencing it, a person may become
more open to the thing itself. (p. 80)

In a paper I wrote entitled, "Unknowing: Toward Another Pattern
of Knowing in Nursing" (1993c), I suggested that this type of activity
is necessary in all our encounters with individuals, whether for research or otherwise. However, the aim of bracketing is to set aside
our own beliefs for a period of time so that we can "hear" and "see,"
as undisturbed as is possible by our own knowing. This unknowing
allows for openness and also allows us to converse with participants
without attempting to validate our own presuppositions and beliefs.
Many of us spend a great deal of time trying to convince others to see
the world the way we do. When they don't, we say they don't understand. In the unknowing stance, however, we say we do not understand and wish to understand other perspectives.

The following passage written by Jane Smiley (1989) describes the
same phenomenon:

As I sit on this hard bench I suddenly yearn for one last long look
and not only of the phenomenon of little Joe and little Michael, but
of the others too; Ellen, four, and Annie, seven months, sharing a
peach. . . . As I watch them now as adults the fact that I will never
see their toddler selves again is tormenting. (p. 120)

Ann Beattie (1989) wrote in a similar vein:

When you are thirty, the child is two. At forty, you realize that
the child in the house, the child you live with, is still, when you
close your eyes, or the moment he has walked from the room, two
years old. When you are sixty and the child is gone, the child will
also be two, but then you will be more certain. Wet sheets, wet
kisses. A flood of tears. As you remember him the child is always
two. (p. 53)

We will now embark on a discussion that is essential to understand if we want to truly grasp the experience of the other. The challenge is to *appreciate different meanings,* as illustrated in the preceding examples.

BRACKETING AS UNKNOWING AND DECENTERING*

Bracketing attempts to achieve the essential state of mind of unknowing as a condition of openness. In contrast, knowing leads to a form of confidence that has inherent in it a state of closure. The "art" of unknowing is discussed as a decentering process from the individual's own organizing principles of the world (Atwood & Stolorow, 1984). Unknowing is not simple, but essential to the understanding of subjectivity and perspectivity.

Unknowing paradoxically is another form of knowing. *Knowing that you do not know something,* that you do not understand someone who stands before you, and who perhaps does not fit into some preexisting paradigm or theory is critical to the evolution of understanding meaning for others.

To engage in an authentic encounter means standing in your own socially constructed world and—in order to unearth the other's world—saying "I do not know you. I do not know your subjective world." A person who engages another human being to form impressions, formulate a perception, and theorize from a place called knowing has confidence in prior knowledge. Such confidence, however, has inherent in it a state of closure. To be authentically present to a person is to situate knowingly in your own life and interact with full unknowingness about the other's life. In this way, unknowing equals openness (see Figure 4.1).

This, by no means, is easy. Unknowing as an art is not presently acknowledged and calls for a great amount of introspection.

---

* Parts of this discussion come from P. L. Munhall, "Unknowing: Toward a Fifth Pattern of Knowing," *Nursing Outlook.* Copyright 1993. Used with permission. May/June 1993, Vol. 41, No. 3.

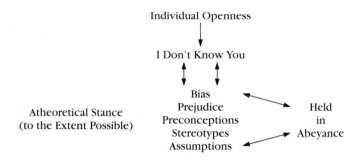

Figure 4.1. Unknowing Openness.

"Unknowing," however, remains essential to the understanding of intersubjectivity and perspectivity. In other words, it is essential to understand ourselves and the participants in our study as two distinctive beings, one of whom the researcher does not know. Each of us has a unique perspective of our situated context and a unique perspective of who we are as individuals in the world. This is our perspectivity, our worldview and our reality. When the researcher and the participant meet, two perspectives of a situation need to be recognized. Thus the process of intersubjectivity begins to create a perceptual space (see Figure 4.2).

Intersubjectivity

Intersubjectivity is not difficult to understand though many writings seem intent on making the concept seem complex. What is complex *is practicing it* in a wide-awake manner.

Intersubjectivity is the verbal and nonverbal interplay between the organized subjective worlds of two people (Paterson & Zderad, 1976, 1990), in which one person's subjectivity intersects with another's subjectivity. The subjective world of any individual represents the organization of feeling, thoughts, ideas, principles, theories, illusions, distortions, and whatever else helps or hinders that person. The real point here is that individuals do not know about anyone else's subjective world unless they are told about it. And even then, they cannot be sure. Figure 4.3 illustrates visually the concepts of intersubjectivity.

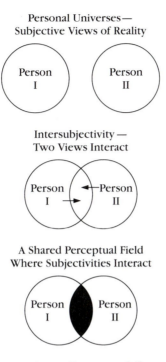

Figure 4.2. Perceptual Space.

So as the researcher begins to converse with the participant, the *researcher does so as the unknower and thinks of the other as the knower.*

The knower tells the researcher, who doesn't know, "what it is like" for that participant. Listening to *the whole story* with prompters is essential before an in-depth dialogue can take place. That is why many interviews with the same person are suggested. The problem of interruptions during the beginning, as I see it, is that interruption itself may lead the interview in another direction and what was to be told may be lost as a result.

As part of this unknowing and interviewing relationship, I suggest that you remain a listener as long as possible, using only prompters such as "Go ahead," "Go on," "Could you tell me more?"

Self enters even when you prompt with "That's interesting, could you tell me more about that?" Most of us want to be interesting so

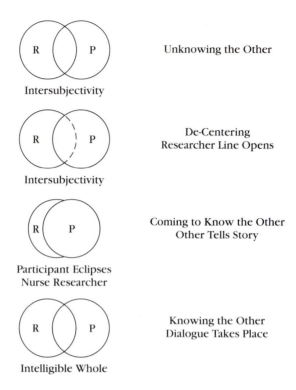

Figure 4.3. Intersubjectivity and the Other.

participants may gladly oblige, but in their reality, what they're saying might not interest them at all. The following suggested formula works for me:

- *Interview 1.* Allow the other to become comfortable speaking with you.
- *Interview 2.* Allow the other to tell his or her story.
- *Interview 3.* Develop dialogic conversation, encouraging other to make interpretation or talk of the meaning of the experience.
- *Interview 4.* Dialogic conversation continues and deepens. Researcher attempts to clarify meanings and asks unknowing questions.

A DECENTERING PROCESS

This art of unknowing when two subjective worlds intersect is discussed as a decentering process, one that decenters us from our own organizing principles of the world (Atwood & Stolorow, 1984). The art of unknowing enables the researcher to know the situated context where it becomes possible to understand the actual essence of meaning that another person finds in an experience.

Figure 4.3 also represents the concept called "being for others," which Sartre thought of utmost importance in understanding and evaluating the human situation. What is portrayed here as decentering is a temporary suspending of self as the research allows the other's subjective structure of reality to become known. The researcher metaphorically is eclipsed by another in order to know the other. The researcher encourages the other to reveal his or her perspective without interruption or the introduction of alternative interpretation. The researcher's respect encourages the participant "to be" seen and heard and furthers deeper understanding.

The proceeding is a possibility, recalling that the phenomenon and situated context are alive in ways that tell us how to proceed. Actually, the word "interview" does not sound very phenomenological to my ear. Asking people to tell their stories and then, at some point, asking for further clarification or meaning (their meaning, not ours) is what we are about. Is an apology in order for sounding Zen? Because we are wedded to the Western mind-set, other ways of thinking often sound desonant. So while it may make individuals feel more at home to say: First you bracket; then you interview; then you do a thematic analysis, extraction, and find meaning units; I say: Be mindful. Practice mindfulness. Does this language sound congruent with phenomenologist philosophy?

Before I hear someone tell their story, I like to think. I think about the art of unknowing and the art of listening. I *really do* try to quiet my own thoughts and absorb the story. Next time you are having a conversation, try not to be thinking of a response. If the person you are speaking with is from the Western mind-set culture, he or she will often finish with "Well, what do you think?"

If you are decentered (hold theories and assumptions in abeyance), you would answer, "Could you tell me more?" You become more knowing and so it goes.

You are in such a place of openness that starting places no longer seem relevant. You are open to all the material depicted in Figure 2.1 and you are aware of all the different ways to enter a house.

Imagination and openness are the essential characteristics. From every place:

Everything beckons to us to perceive it. (Rilke, p. 10)

I haven't told you about Chuck and Ray recently. I am trying to decenter myself in telling of this most recent turn of events. Intersubjectivity is so critical that I have asked them to do a narrative about this experience for a later chapter.

But for now, I'd like to let you know that Chuck has accepted a position as Chairperson of a Nursing Department in New Hampshire. In fact, I met him at yet another airport (Newark for that matter), where he was flying off for the interview and I was flying back to Miami. At that time, neither of us thought he would actually move. More to come.

5

We Laughed a Little, We Cried a Little
Personal Experience in Phenomenology

This chapter presents personal experience as having an affective and emotional component in its telling. Telling your story can be emotionally cathartic. Hearing others' stories can raise your level of sensitivity and contribute enormously to your understanding of other perceptions and ways of being in an experience.

However, the idea of "readiness" must be considered. Phenomenology as a research approach may assist us in better understanding an experience, but it should not be used in an effort to resolve conflicts about personal issues. We may have had the experience under study, or be close to it; yet it is essential to evaluate the readiness to study the phenomenon. Sometimes, it may be blurry because we cannot predict, but we should be clear as to the purpose of the study; resolution of conflicts is not an acceptable one! Personal problems may be unintentionally resolved as a bonus, but the waters will be murky if controversy exists at the start.

Personal experience, however, is an essential part of a phenomenological study. Somehow, in some way, we are related to the experience and that needs to be explored and told about. We also know that this material is only one part of the study and often contains elements that we need to put aside temporarily in order to become the unknower.

---

*I*n the previous chapters, we discussed personal experience as a starting point, but here I want to talk about the affective and emotive potential of phenomenology for caring in the pursuit of understanding the meaning of being. For many years, this value was not considered the domain of science and therefore was not appropriate to study; now it seems to have slipped into the life-world of education. Having had the privilege of teaching courses and seminars on phenomenology, I have come to understand how ingrained this attitude has become.

I mention this here for a few reasons. If you are a teacher, researcher, or student, you need to reflect on your own level within the affective emotive domain of coming to understand through all the senses. If you are a researcher or student and describing your own experience is emotional for you or if a human experience that you wish to understand better has moved you to tears, then you must also evaluate your capacity for self-revelation and the display of emotion. Again, *readiness* must be considered.

In the following example, Patricia, one of my students, wanted to describe her experience of being childless because of an early hysterectomy. She wanted to present this in class and was quite confident that she could do so. What she discovered—and this is very important—was that she felt much more comfortable speaking about someone else's experience. So she did that first, and then tearfully she read her own. There was not a dry eye in the class. I'll speak more to that later, but first I will present some of the experiences that were brought forth.

The First Experience

In order to get to her own experience, Patricia first asked another individual to describe her experience. Because phenomenology starts with the personal does not necessarily mean that a researcher must write a description of his or her own experience before doing anything else. In attempting to be naive before interviewing individuals, this initial step is important, but in other instances, first learning about another person's experience can be liberating.

Steps again may seem out of order when a phenomenon appears to you and you are trying to begin to understand it; then you realize there is a research opportunity before you. As the process unfolded for Patricia, another individual first wrote this story at her request:

I Would Have Liked to Have Had a Child

When I was first asked to write a story about my situation, I thought to myself that it should be pretty easy since I can still remember everything as if it was yesterday. Then I started to write it all down on paper and things were not quite so easy. My first question was "How do I explain to complete strangers what my surgery meant to me and how it affected me emotionally?" With this in mind, I have tried starting this story about 6 times, each time to no avail, and the paper only ending up in the trash can. Then I decided that it might be easier to just write it on my computer so that I could make changes as I go. I quickly learned how to cut and paste paragraphs and pages in Wordperfect. By now you have guessed that I am very nervous in talking about my surgery. Suddenly, I have written a whole page just on the introduction and have not gotten into the story yet. So here goes!!

As you can tell from the title, this is my story of how I would have liked to have a child, but no longer have the opportunity to bear children. I had to have a hysterectomy just a little over a year ago due to medical reasons. This might appear to be not such a big deal because at least now I have my health to be thankful for but somehow that just doesn't make it any easier to accept. I am 36 years old and have never been married. I just have not found the right guy to settle down with and have a family. Therefore the idea of having a child was put on the back burner until I got married (of course the age-old school of thought that you should be married to have a child).

Well, a few years back I started having spells of vertigo followed by migraine headaches. The vertigo spells were at the start of the headaches. I think I was afraid of the spells themselves because I never knew when they might occur.

My gynecologist started me on Lupron shots monthly to see if the migraine headaches occurred. The final result was that I needed a total hysterectomy to stop the headaches and vertigo spells. I made the decision to have the surgery because I had 3 full months without a headache or spell and it felt wonderful to be back to my old self again. Little did I realize that I had not even thought of how the surgery was going to affect me emotionally after all was said and done.

I really didn't think about the fact that I couldn't have any children until after I had recovered physically from the surgery. I remember the first time I had a nightmare about it. I cried for a while after I woke up because I felt like I had been stripped of the chance to have my own child. *I realized I could never become a natural parent or a grandparent. I would never be able to give my parents a grandchild even though I knew that they were grandparents for both my brothers' children. I just felt that I couldn't and didn't want to accept that this had happened to me. Sure the headaches and the vertigo finally stopped about six months after the surgery, but what a price I felt that I had paid for a normal life. Was it worth giving up the opportunity to have a child to have pain-free, carefree life?*

For months I thought I had made the wrong decision. I just couldn't come to terms with it. I avoided all my friends with children because I couldn't face it. I felt cheated. Why did this happen to me? What did I do to deserve it? I love children and always have. I began wanting something I could never have. During this time I had terrible mood swings and tried to find fault with everything and everyone. Nothing satisfied me. I began to hurt the people that really cared to me and didn't appreciate their help or support. I just felt like they wouldn't understand because I couldn't understand it myself. I didn't want to hear what anyone said because I didn't want to discuss it. My solution was to avoid the issue and it would go away. But unfortunately it just gets buried deeper and makes things worse.

I had a serious argument with the dearest and closest people to me. I felt like I had lost and betrayed the people who are here now and love me for what I am. I took a long look at my life as it was and felt that I was pretty lucky to be healthy. Because of the surgery, I was able to get back to a normal, active life. I really began to be thankful for what was and not depressed over what wasn't.

I realized that it was not out the realms of possibility of marrying into a ready-made family one of these days. I have nieces and 2 godchildren whom I love to spoil and spend time with. Maybe someday, I might even be in a position to adopt a child (God knows there are plenty of children who need good homes). Sure I will know in my mind that it is not my natural child but in my heart that won't matter.

Having a hysterectomy is not the end of the world for a single female as I felt at first. It just happened to be one of life's many obstacles. I am not saying that I am completely over it emotionally, but maybe just able to accept it a little easier. Thank you for listening even though I am not here to tell it. I hope that maybe it will help you to understand a little more the next time you hear of a female who has had surgery. The best gift you could give them would be your support, your shoulder, and time. Doctors and nurses support the physical healing, but friends and family support the emotional healing.

Thanks very much, Pat, for asking me to do this. I am sure now you knew it would help me, which it definitely has [emphasis added].

Patricia's Experience

After sharing that experience, Patricia was then able to write her own personal experience. Other personal experiences of students in the class followed. Only students who wanted to share personal experiences did so. A person does not have to have the experience in order to study it; however, a researcher does begin with personal experience in which his or her relatedness to the phenomenon under study is described.

Patricia introduced her experience with a quotation.

The poet Rilke describes how lived experience, memory, time, and reflections are all involved in writing:

> *One must have memories . . . and still it is not yet enough to have memories. One must be able to forget them when they are many and we must have the great patience to wait until they come again. For it is not yet the memories themselves. Not till they have turned to look within us, to glance and gesture, nameless and no longer to be distinguished from ourselves— not till then can it happen that in some most rare hour the first word of a verse arises in their midst and goes forth from them.*

What is it like to be childless?

Help Me to Understand

All your life you grow up dreaming and wondering of what your spouse and children will be like. Will I have a boy or a girl or maybe both? Will they look like me, will they be bright and above all will they be healthy?

This fantasy begins when we as very young girls begin playing with dolls. We begin the formation of nurturing, playing mother and the need to "practice for the future." Our society lends itself to following the norm of growing up, getting married, and having a family.

That norm was altered for me. After many years of multiple gynecological problems and experiencing every treatment that existed to humankind, it came to an end five years ago when I almost hemorrhaged to death. The most forbidden word "hysterectomy" was suggested to me as the only alternative left. At that moment a cold chill, an emptiness filled my heart. I experienced a feeling I will never be able to totally explain. The surgery was successful and I have healed postoperatively beautifully, but emotional scars still exist. There are many times that I want to scream and holler and ask, "Why me?" "Why was I robbed of my motherhood?"

My mother and I are best friends and I have always wanted a little girl to share the same kind of gift we share. I am reminded every day of my inability to be a natural mother. The little baby in church that clings to his mother for security, or the TV commercials advertising diapers or baby food, or the patients that ask me how many children I have, and finally the baby showers that I avoid because it reminds me of my loss.

I will never feel that special bond of a child that is shared between a husband and a wife. I will never hear those tiny footsteps on the kitchen floor, the gurgling and cooing of my babies as they lie in their crib, or the cry to be fed at 3:00 A.M. I will miss their first footsteps, their first words, and their first day at school.

"Why me?" "Why was motherhood taken out of my life plan?" I have always loved children, and I always thought I would be a good Mom. I see older patients that have no children; their spouses have died and they are so alone. They suffer such misery and such solitude. I also see some women who conceive at the blink of an eye and then I see child abuse. It's not fair.

Is it selfish for me to feel like this? To want to share love and happiness with a child that is an extension of me, or for my children to know the wonderful grandparents or uncle they would have had?

I am learning to deal with the ache in my heart. Yes, there is adoption, and maybe some day this will be an option for me, but for now I still need to accept and understand "why me?"

Patricia Hurst (1992)

Patricia told her experience movingly, but she said she was not yet able to study it further. She did say, however, that this was very beneficial to her and that in some way she felt stronger and perhaps able to study it in the future.

Another Experience

The following personal experience, described by Vivian Sanchez (1992), shows a similar human response:

What is it like to experience a miscarriage? I remember sitting on the emergency room table thinking, How could this be happening to me? It just isn't so. These things don't happen to me. I could not concentrate on anything while I waited for my doctor to arrive. The room, the situation was so unfamiliar to me. I did not like being there—I wished I were home. I was taken to the sonogram room, and everyone was so silent when the procedure was being done. I tried to smile and let them think I was strong, I was OK and that I could deal with it. I was shocked by the news 30 minutes later that there was no heartbeat. The fetus had died. I was in disbelief and then the anger came. I wanted the dead tissues out of my body, almost in repulsion of the entire situation. I remember seeing the visible signs of the impending miscarriage as I waited for a D&C. I could not think of waiting an entire day to let the tissues pass naturally. I wanted it out. As I waited, a tremendous sadness filled me. A kind nurse told me it was OK to cry because I was experiencing a loss. All I could think of was that loss. After the procedure, I felt a bewildering emptiness like I had never felt before. My first loss, I call this.

Months have passed, and I still recall the emotions I felt that day in the emergency room, and if I'm alone and thinking to myself, I cringe with sadness and hurt still. Songs I hear on the radio recall my loss; the clothes I wore that day recall it. I think of it often, sometimes too often.

This is a lived experience description, not a phenomenological description, but from it I sense that there is a meaning of the experience for me. In an effort to cope with this experience, before ever studying phenomenology, I talked to people who had miscarriages and read books written by women who had experienced the same thing. I was trying to understand the situation to find common ground with others who had experienced the same things. Indeed, now that I have studied phenomenology and its quest to find meaning in the lived experience, I believe my research question can be, "What is it like to experience a miscarriage?" Perhaps I'm still too emotional about its impact on me personally, but with time I feel it is a valid phenomenological research question that could shed light on this experience. Indeed, what I did find was that women commonly do experience loss, depression, and a lessening of self-esteem.

A research study to explore the meaning of miscarriage has great implications for nursing practice. The study could help nurses become more human, more sensitive to the needs of women. Indeed, the experience transformed me and the transformation has brought me to a heightened attentiveness and thoughtfulness to this experience, which phenomenology requires one to do. It also has given me a sense of participation in the world. As a phenomenologist doing research, one is also asked to participate in one's research question.

Vivian realized through this sharing that she was not ready to study this phenomenon. This reluctance is important to consider and respect.

READINESS

If the researcher, as in the foregoing example, is very emotionally sensitive, I usually suggest not researching that particular experience until a later time. Frequently, I have had students who seem to want to work through their own suffering or pain. If this approach worked, I would be supportive of such an idea. However, in my own experience with such situations, students seemingly must first attain a certain perceptible level of resolution or acceptance of the experience.

I have learned this from many years of advising students who seem often to pursue a phenomenological question that pertains to their own being in the world. They have been there. I think there are ways of ascertaining readiness to study a lived experience that have to do with the resolution of the conflicts brought about by the experience.

It can be difficult to determine the level of acceptance that the student or researcher has reached, but if the person is tearful all the time, choked up when speaking about the phenomenon, or has a voice tone that conveys pain, then I believe it is not yet the time to do this phenomenological study.

My aim is not necessarily to discourage a subjective study (although that is a serious consideration) but more to emphasize that phenomenology is not intended to resolve the emotional conflicts of the researcher. If and when the temporal and relational dimensions change for Vivian, she might be able to do a fine study on experiencing a miscarriage. To say that the researcher needs to achieve some distance might sound paradoxical when the goal is to understand what it is to be human, yet this distance is not linear but emotional. This limitation ensures that the researcher does not suffer or contribute to others' suffering.

A good example, in addition to Vivian's own recognition, is another student, who wanted to describe her personal experience of having a mastectomy. I did not think she was ready to do so in a public way, but she insisted she was able. I discouraged her and let her know my concerns. But she told me that she wanted to tell her story. When the time came for her to do so, however, her own personal insight that very night was that she was not ready to share her experience. It was too painful.

I felt this student's pain and understood her suffering. Because her experience was so much with her, I also realized she could not unknow herself well with others. I did not believe she could interview other women in ways that would allow unknowing to be mindful.

Whether we are in the role of student or teacher, sometimes the better action is to be a health care professional and let the therapeutic imperative override the research imperative by suggesting ways individuals can seek help. Over the years, I have often found that this is what some students are seeking when they come to talk about their research interest.

What we choose to research, in one way or another, reveals who we are, even if the revealing is one of concealing. As I said in an earlier chapter, I am a woman; I like research when it is phenomenologically oriented. As a female researcher, I am interested in many things that affect women. I am sure my research emphasis on women's emotions tells a lot about me. My work on anger as experientially lived by women reveals a value I attach to the emotion and have indeed felt. I went toward it to study when I was ready to—not before, or when I had "somewhat" resolved the way I was with anger—but when I came to recognize that it was as an OK way to be at times, and that recognizing and verbalizing anger could be helpful for women.

So readiness needs to be evaluated, and our criterion of reasonableness is part of that discussion.

The following example is from a student whose personal experience is not distant from her but is integrated into her being in such a way as to enhance her. As a result, she is able to seek further understanding of this phenomenon. She has altruistic as well as personal motives for her study. She wishes, when she was growing up, she had understood what she does now. Yet, she is not doing a case study. She is also aware that others may have different experiences with her situated context, and she is able to give them voice as well.

Robin Parker (1992) related this personal experience:

Experiential Context of Study

The experiential context which this researcher will bring to the study of this phenomenon will influence the researcher's understanding of what it means to parent an ADHD [attention-deficit hyperactivity disorder] child. If a researcher is able to present an accurate history of her/his experience(s) with coming to understand the phenomenon under study, the researcher can then also begin to recognize the layers of interpreted meaning related to the phenomenon that have developed within the researcher's perceptions. This experiential awareness can be a useful technique in beginning to set aside (bracket) the layers of interpretation, so that the phenomenon of interest is seen, as if for the very first time, through the eyes, perceptions, and experiences of the participants.

The researcher's interest in the study of parenting an ADHD child has been influenced by life, education, and career experiences.

Presenting the experiential context in the first-person voice will allow the reader to enter the world of the researcher and hopefully experience where the researcher is coming from prior to the beginning of this study's data collection phase. Therefore, the researcher, henceforth identified in the first-person context, will highlight experiences perceived to influence my interest in this phenomenon. These influences will include my personal experiences, my undergraduate and graduate education, and a description of how I was influenced by my graduate professors.

I was powerfully influenced by my younger brother's ADHD. I was 4 years old when he was born. He was a very attractive child with blonde hair, blue eyes, and a beautiful smile. As the poem by Susan Hughes (1990) pointed out, you couldn't tell by looking at him that he had "something wrong inside." That something was ADHD. His childhood was hard on all of us, but particularly so for my brother and my parents. As a teenager, I was frequently asked to baby-sit my brother; this was a disaster for both of us. My parents tried many interventions; almost nothing worked. The primary emotions, as I remember from my parents when dealing with my brother's ADHD symptoms were anger, fear, and a sense of failure. My brother did not receive the parenting he needed because I believe that my parents did not receive the support they so desperately needed to help guide them in caring for and parenting my brother. I remember my parents' anger and frustration when the physicians provided conflicting information on the cause of ADHD and how to handle the resulting problems. As a result, my brother and parents were often left to struggle through this experience in pain and for the most part alone. I began to wonder, what could help my family? The questions at this stage in the evolution of this study became: What could improve the quality of life for families with children like my brother?

Within the context of this study, it is important to discuss how I became interested in nursing as a career and professional choice. At a very early age, I began to experience severe allergic reactions. These illness episodes would manifest themselves as recurrent anaphylaxis shock. In addition, I developed hyperactive airway disease (asthma). The anaphylaxis shock and the asthma resulted in numerous emergency room visits, and hospitalizations. At a very early age, I experienced the comfort, compassion, and caring expressed to me by the nurses in these hospitals. The nurses cared for me when I was frightened, lonely, and sick. These early experiences influenced my decision to be a nurse. At five, I decided I was going to be a nurse, and I never changed my mind. I know that nursing was the right profession for me; that was 32 years ago, and I have never regretted my decision.

In the researcher's undergraduate ADN program, technical proficiency was the goal. As a nursing student, I worked very hard to memorize tremendous amounts of materials and took frequent multiple-choice exams. During my two years in this program, there was no mention of nursing theory, nursing research (specifically phenomenology), or emphasis on nursing care from the patient's need perspective. Instead, I remember the emphasis being placed on designing plans of care based on the nursing process. In this program, for the most part, the instructors did not allow me the luxury of questioning the curriculum and course design, assignments, and/or the purpose of many learning experiences. I remember feeling intimidated and fearing my instructors would single me out as an example of "something done wrong." Instructors reminded students on a regular basis that "you can be excused from this program right up until the day you graduate." All learning situations and exams were designed to help us pass State Boards exams. With regard to that, we all did very well. I was not encouraged to pursue any further education or advanced practice degree.

During my graduate studies in nursing, I have been drawn to three professors who demonstrated a compassionate sensitivity to my learning needs, while encouraging self-directed scholarly inquiry. The specialness of these three professors arose out of their ability to combine the serious graduate study experience with individuality, humor, and patience. These professors were and are confident enough in their own self-image to encourage me to disagree with them, thereby allowing me to challenge and change my own worldview. These three professors extend themselves and their energies way beyond the usual student-faculty relationships. They are humanistic, compassionate, genuine, and caring; yet at the same time, they are academic leaders and nursing scholars in their service to students, patients, and families and society.

Each of these three nursing professors has influenced and motivated me to continue with the exploration and investigation needed for this study. They have served as professional role models to me, and have motivated me to study nursing. I am fortunate to be able to state that they are my thesis committee and will help guide this study. As each of them has significantly influenced my development as well as this study's development over the course of the past two years, I felt it was important to share this as a part of my experiential context.

We can see from this personal account one way an individual reveals and conceals. Robin is studying the meaning of being a parent of a hyperactive child. We could, if we wished to, psychoanalyze this way of going about understanding what it is like to be a sister of a hyperactive child.

Van Manen said once (Summer Workshop, 1992) that psychoanalysis fills in where phenomenology leaves questions. But it is important, I think, to understand that unless a person is a phenomenological psychoanalyst, this inquiry would place Robin's study under unnecessary scrutiny. Her research is just fine and I believe it will make a valuable contribution to our understanding of this way of being.

SOME IMPORTANT POINTS ABOUT PERSONAL EXPERIENCE

First, as I already said and now am demonstrating, there is repetition in this text. I believe in repetition. So I am taking my own subjective notion and projecting it to my readers. Some of you may object, even silently complain, thinking *she already said that;* and then again, some of you will be glad to be reminded. I repeat the points I want to emphasize.

I have been telling you about my friends Chuck and Ray during the course of this book, to illustrate the everydayness of the concepts in phenomenology. In Chapter 1, I told you about abandonment. At the same time, I discussed consciousness and the need to be careful of the unconscious, which can be very unruly; if we're not aware of its potential effects, we may forever be acting in ways we are not aware of.

This is what my unconscious did today:

Chuck and Ray, who are definitely now moving to New Hampshire and leaving me here in Miami, have been gone for a week. They asked if I would take care of their two dogs for the week. I did not relish the idea; after all, there are two of them to split the care and only one of me—and the dogs are quite a handful. Well, it's the sixth day, and as I write, I am hoping both dogs are recovering from heat stroke.

It was hot, muggy, and noonish. I took them for a walk. I was not aware of the weather, I seldom am down here except, it seems, for hurricanes. I thought the dogs would really like a nice long walk. Unconscious to the temperature, and the sun, off we went with my best intentions. It was Saturday, I had been writing and needed a break. Well, one mile into the walk, one of the dogs decided to lie down. This had never happened before. I gave him a slight tug, and the other one collapsed, too. I realized I knew nothing about these dogs, but obviously they could not tolerate the heat. What was I doing? I was perspiring from the heat and from the anxiety of the reality—now fully blown out of proportion—that my unconscious wanted to get rid of these dogs (I was counting the days). I carried the dogs home. Now, for the past two hours and after two phone calls to other dog-knowledgeable friends (Chuck and Ray have no number to be reached at), I have worried about nothing else. I don't remember the dog I had when I lived up North acting this way.

Now they are up and about and I am just amazed at how the unconscious works. So while we have paid due attention to consciousness in phenomenology, the preceding anecdote demonstrates the following important ideas relative to phenomenological studies:

1. My assumptions, presuppositions, were wrong.
2. Apparently, unconscious anger was acted out, though consciously I thought I was being generous.
3. I did not consider my situated context—the size of the dogs, the time of day, the temperature, north versus south, and all of us in our bodies.
4. From one anecdote, themes emerge: failure of good intentions, danger of lack of knowledge, fear for animals, recognition of possible unconscious motivation, admission of being wrong, and relief the dogs seemed all right.

This is an example of what can go into a journal. What's important is that the experience is with me; I am very present to it. Writing in a journal when the experience is still fresh is a good habit to get into during your study. Stories are never finished or never told completely. What if I were to add the following true information?

1. The dogs felt abandoned in a strange place—at least they acted angry.
2. They were totally incontinent for the entire time even though they were walked 3 times a day.
3. They barked at night and kept me awake.
4. They chewed up some of my shoes and clothes.

5. At night, Chuck and Ray called to ask how the dogs were.
6. I did not tell Chuck and Ray all that was happening.

Now we do further exploration. That is why I suggest many interviews. In this example, the following meanings can now be understood:

1. Situated context is certainly enlarged in terms of space and time, relationality, and embodiment.
2. I was experiencing frustration.
3. As caretaker, I was in a state of sleep deprivation.
4. Chuck and Ray really were not at fault, but really?

When I told my friend Virginia about this situation the first night, she said I should put the dogs in a kennel and pick them up before picking up Chuck and Ray at the airport. I now know that how people react to this entire saga will be completely subjective. Dog lovers perhaps won't understand and will think me a poor sport (my own self-criticism during the entire episode).

Add another item to the list: self-criticism—I should be doing better.

There is a complete phenomenological text here. Also, the everydayness of life can never be overestimated as far as its effects. It just is not as simple as leaving two dogs with a friend. And people outside the experience would probably think of it as an ordinary life event. But it wasn't. It could have had a tragic ending.

My dog-sitting experience also reminds us that assumptions are critical in understanding human behavior, the role played by projection, and the necessity of bracketing or unknowing in the study of lived experience. Projection refers to the belief that others think and feel the same way we do. We believe they share our assumptions about reality. Often, with this maneuver, we hear a person accusing others of something the person actually does but is blind to. In this example, the presumed intersubjective conjunction is: If we love our dogs, then you too will love our dogs. In our research activities, we have to be careful to identify our subjective structure of reality.

Interviews or dialogues or whatever we choose to call the way we seek understanding should not be an effort to produce evidence that confirms our perception of an experience.

The study of experiences is *not to substantiate our perceptions.* In fact, a good study just might *liberate us from our preconceptions.* This is why we become introspective about the phenomenon or our beliefs about a specific experience. To follow this again with the dogs (the darlings), my preconception about this week had to do with reattaching to a pet, since I had long had one. I assured Chuck and Ray, "Everything will be fine . . . we all know that at the end of the week, I'll be out getting myself a dog . . . since all dog owners [projecting] think I'll be much happier with one."

With nine hours to go, my prediction was waning. The supposed pleasures of having a pet don't seem to apply to me right now in my life-world (although it might change). However, I'm still stuck with self-criticism, as if something is wrong with me. From a psychological orientation, there is surely more to this than what is being said. The present text is on phenomenology not psychology, and yet it is easy to see how closely they are linked. This is why psychologists and now psychoanalysts have developed research methods from the philosophy of phenomenology.

There will be much discussion on interviewing, but I think, at this juncture, it is evident that projection prevents the researcher from hearing the other with clarity. Literally, leave your beliefs at home and find out how others structure their reality, how others perceive their world; be truly unknowing so that you can be open to variations and even contradictions of your cherished beliefs. Such discoveries *do not* mean you are wrong; they tell us about alternative meanings of experiences. Validity in a phenomenological study is just that: the unaltered faithful telling of experiences by people.

I don't think we can ever overestimate the importance of the situated context. It is all—the critical variable, so to speak, that often is not mentioned except as categories. Not only is the situated context the all, it really becomes the "all" only after someone has told you about it. Situated contexts conjure up assumptions, but the researcher must question, What meaning does the context have? How does it weave into the experience being studied? How is this context interpreted by the human involved?

For example, a woman related to me:

I am 40 years old, have 2 children ages 6 years and 10 years. I quit my job 10 years ago because my husband moved around a lot due to his job. I have devoted myself to his career and our children, which worked out well. The other day he comes home and tells me he is leaving, for another woman. He said he's sorry and tells me I should get an attorney and his attorney will work out the details.

Say that's all you know. What is your reaction? What is your interpretation? What are possible preconceptions and assumptions? I could reply after hearing this:

"That's terrible."

"How horrible, how will you manage?"

"The _____. You gave him everything and then he leaves at his convenience."

"It just goes to show, you should not quit your job."

All those replies, however, if I did say that, would represent projection. Instead, I proceed unknowingly as is proper in a phenomenological study (and ironically also in the practice of psychotherapy) and say, "Could you tell me more?"

She replies:

First, of course, I was shocked and angry, but as I began to reflect on it over a week or so, I began to feel a cloud over me pass on. I wasn't even aware of this cloud, I wasn't even aware of being. I guess I had lost myself in many ways. I thought I loved Jack and maybe I still do but I was living my life for him. This might not last, but right now I feel he just gave me a big present. I have my life back. I know I shouldn't feel this way (herself know a victim of assumptions) but I feel positively optimistic. Is that crazy?

I thought to myself as regards this phenomenological approach, it is so wonderful to see old myths and assumptions challenged in this way. Remember, however, to keep your research role prominent, unless this is a clinical description for your study; keep the research perspective in front of you: the meaning of being human, this experience perhaps of being the party to a divorce.

The next response then would be (again not very different than psychotherapy): "I'm not sure what you mean by crazy?" Most likely, her response will be based on preconceptions, assumptions, and well-ingrained myths about how she *should* feel. Feeling different from the learned should, she questions her sanity.

An important justification for doing studies from the perspective of situated contexts is that they include an individual's interpretations and can lead to different ways to understand the experience. The dilemmas raised by AIDS (acquired immuno-deficiency syndrome) provide another example. All our theories, beliefs, and assumptions about grief, even the stages of grieving, are in flux and being questioned in the tragedy of the AIDS epidemic. Grieving seems to be different from the agreed-on version of the process. It's bad enough to be grieving but even worse if you feel you're not doing it right or not according to the strictures of some theory. This type of going back, opening up, allowing other to be different, rather than deviant, is the promise that phenomenology offers to us. How could we think otherwise? Depending on the context, the meaning of being human in situations will vary greatly. We will not think of people as being noncompliant but as experiencing their being in a different way. The meaning of their experience needs our attentiveness.

Attentiveness needs to be part of what we do when we embark on phenomenological studies. Thus far, we have discussed attentiveness to intersubjectivity, the role of personal experience and readiness to study a particular human experience, as well as attentiveness to our unconscious. Reflection is critical to all these processes.

6

I Can Hear Clearly Now
Interviews, Conversations, and Writing

This chapter introduces notions and ideas concerning phenomenological interviews and conversations. Discussion includes interviews from clinical practice, volunteer interviews, and "technique" questions that students are concerned about.

Concrete examples of what can be created from interviews and mindfulness are presented to show how a researcher arrives at thematic statements and essential themes, and then through linguistic transformation is able to write a phenomenological study. However, you always need to be wary of the slippery slope of techniques and formulas, lest they become a stronger focus than the study of meaning.

Although the term "dialogic conversation" implies a redundancy, I find it useful in distinguishing such interchanges from social conversations. The real dialogue comes from the storyteller; the prompter of the dialogue is the "unknower," the researcher.

This chapter, like an outline, is intended to set forth the concrete, "how to" part of phenomenology. I think of these techniques as a way for beginners in the area to become more comfortable, not necessarily more phenomenological.

But if our heart is not with them, their previous presence is neglected, and they no longer exist. We must be aware of them to ap-

preciate their value. . . . If through carelessness and forgetfulness
we become dissatisfied with them, and begin asking too much . . .
we will lose them.

Thich Nhat Hanh
(1988, p. 90)

Van Manen (1990) states:

> *In hermeneutic phenomenological human science the interview*
> *serves very specific purposes: (1) it may be used as a means for ex-*
> *ploring and gathering experiential narrative material that may*
> *serve as a resource for developing a richer and deeper understand-*
> *ing of a human phenomenon and (2) the interview may be used as*
> *a vehicle to develop a conversational relation with a partner (inter-*
> *viewee) about the meaning of an experience. (p. 66)*

While the interview provides us with critical phenomenological
material, I think it is essential to understand that existential investigation of a phenomenon is *not limited* to interviews with people
who are willing to talk about something. The interview, however, as
a dialogic conversation, is an extremely important part of our attempt to understand a person in a practice setting or a group of individuals in a research endeavor.

BASIC INFORMATION ABOUT INTERVIEWS

In our evolution over the past ten years or so, our studies from the
phenomenological method have often relied primarily on interviews.
Researchers often performed the following activities and asked the
following questions or made such observations:

1. What questions should I ask?
2. How many people do I need to interview?
3. I can't seem to keep people focused.
4. What do I do with all this material (transcripts)?

First, we must be careful in framing our question. The "what is it
like" approach is fine, understandable and concrete. Asking people to

tell you about their lived experience of *being* cared for might prompt different responses than asking what it is like to *feel* cared for, the phenomenon discussed in Lucy Warren's study (Chapter 15).

Because of their finite difference, I find dialogue important. Any examples, stories, anecdotes, pictures, and writing the individual may be willing to share with you will enrich your study. Along with this, I find the idea of a dialogue to be one of a relationship between two human beings. In this type of conversation, the unknower is seeking understanding of the other speaker and *not* vice versa. Interviewing from this perspective, we see that the intent is different. It is not a demographic interview and, though often tempting, it does not seek reaffirmation of your beliefs. Researchers sometimes find themselves saying:

- Don't you think . . . ?
- Did you find that . . . ?
- Do you think it was because they were . . . ?

Such questions may appear to be harmless, but they have the potential to structure a person's story. The following lead-ins help explicate the person's unfolding of the experience.

- Could you give me an example of that?
- Do you remember how that made you feel (assuming there's a reason for a feeling question)?
- What did that do for you?
- What do you think is the meaning of (whatever preceded)?
- (Or after a sentence) Go on . . . Could you elaborate more on that?

One student told me that her mouth was sore from smiling (remember Gretchen?). While you might smile, this is certainly not a requisite and sometimes would be inappropriate. Try to *follow the mood of the person* you are interviewing. Also be aware of the body, the posture, the intonation in words and the being of the other. Since the interview has sometimes assumed preeminence in the phenomenological approach, other considerations need to be taken:

- If you have never interviewed people before in the form of a dialogic conversation, then you need to practice. Practice with someone who has a background in psychiatric nursing, psychology, or psychoanalysis. In their disciplines, listening is elevated to an art. In phenomenology, listening also becomes an art.

- Listening is an art. Try just to hear what is being said. Try not to be anticipating what comes next—let there be pauses and silence.

- Silence is important. An individual said something. You listen. There is a pause. You are both reflecting. Let the other person break the silence. The pause will often yield additional reflection. Becoming comfortable with a silent or pregnant pause enables the storyteller to probe deeper within. Let it be quiet until you intuit that a prompter might be helpful.

- Many studies are a result of one-time interviews. As I have suggested, two to three interviews with the same person may be more helpful. More "reflected upon" material is usually forthcoming, and you have a chance to mutually agree on the description and interpretation of what was said in previous interviews. A practitioner or researcher who ends a single interview with "Is there anything else you might like to add?" is asking the question for that moment. Often, during the week that follows, more reflection occurs and the person desires to tell more about the experience.

- Imagine yourself in the interviewee's place for the first time. What might he or she be thinking about? Another reason I strongly recommend additional interviews is that there is so much to process in the first encounter. Depending on what you're discussing, you may need to use the first interview to establish trust and rapport. That effort will ensure the integrity of the material forthcoming.

- Be aware of your participant's holistic condition. You do not need to stop an interview if crying or anger takes place (as long as the interviewer knows very well if this is therapeutic). However, you need good judgment. Even though informed consent assures that the interviewee can stop the interview at any time, sometimes the interviewer needs to recognize it is time to relax and change direction. Relief time, perhaps a little casual talk, may be comforting. Our intention here is not psychotherapy or nursing intervention. Our role must be clearly known, and we must act accordingly.

So we need to be cognizant and attuned to our participant's psychological condition. Again, follow-up interviews help protect the psychological comfort of interviewees and demonstrate our genuine interest in them as persons.

Interviews Originating from Clinical Practice

Practicing professionals have access to some interviews in clinical settings that are actual descriptions of lived experiences (see Newman's Research as Praxis).

I personally prefer to call these interviews clinical experiential descriptions. The potential for a study of a phenomenon often becomes apparent in a retrospective way. For example, a nurse has worked three years in a rehabilitation setting for drug or alcohol abuse. Patients tell their stories of what it was like for them. She collects such material from her clinical practice, and perhaps she begins to grasp what this is about—the being-in-the-world of this experience. Often, it is the very involvement in the experience—being within it—that prompts a health care practitioner to see an experience afresh. Can she go back? For a start, she can explain to her patients that their experiences would be valuable in a study she would like to do. She can then discuss her ideas and thoughts with and ask clients or patients to become part of her study.

This process is analogous to the way I have written this book. I was teaching a course on research from a phenomenological perspective when it occurred to me that my students were writing wonderful phenomenological material that would fit well into a text. I asked for permission to use—with proper attribution of authorship—some of their material, and readers will come across these contributions throughout the text.

Also analogous to this is my own research. Much comes from, and originates in, my clinical practice as a nurse psychoanalyst. I do not approach patients as research projects, but I am always informed by them. I cannot separate my concern and curiosity of the nature of being from my own being and their own being and becoming. However, (and researchers do not do this in all fields) I ask patients for permission to use their descriptions of experiences for a study I may be doing. These requests are always retrospective; patients have been telling their stories, and at some point, I begin to understand their experience—what it is like for them. If I think that this insight might contribute to others' understanding of a phenomenon, I might consider researching it. Again, it is extremely important to realize that not all phenomena can be studied in the same way. That is why I say that the phenomenon itself, if we are attuned and become part of it, will show us how to study it.

The discoveries that the researcher makes and the understandings that are communicated in writing are of primary importance. If the study is a good one, we ask, "How did you find this out?" Thus, we are simultaneously developing ways of knowing that recall Feyerbend's question, "Is method antithetical to creativity?"

I have already suggested, as have others, that a method limits us and there is nothing sacred about method prospectively. To know prospectively how to study a phenomenon is to say we already know a lot about it. That itself is actually justification for experimental research. We dare to do experiments because we know or have specific knowledge.

Phenomenology lays no such claim. The "method" is to be as unrestricted and creative as possible in an intense search to understand human experience. In general then, the clinical interview and conversation is one means to achieve understanding and it is indeed an important one. So more suggestions should be considered if they seem appropriate to your situation.

Interviews with Volunteers

This particular section refers to interviews with people who have experienced the phenomenon you wish to understand and have volunteered to share their perceptions with you.

Although it may seem as if the only requirements for interviewing are that the person (1) has had the experience and (2) is willing to speak about it, I think it is important to place *readiness* as a priority condition (see discussion in Chapter 5). While there may be no apparent issue of coercion or expectations, individuals often genuinely wish to be helpful or even feel obligated to consent to an interview without realizing it is not in their best interest. As a researcher, you need to ascertain whether a person is ready emotionally and psychologically for an interview or conversation about his or her experience.

If, when planning your study, you decide that two, three, or four interviews with each person may be necessary for you to acquire an in-depth understanding of the experience as it is understood by the other, then that time requirement also needs to enter the criteria for selection of volunteers. Ideally, interviewees should find that the dialogic conversations help them find understanding, even though that is not a stated purpose. Because of this, between our conversations I have asked persons to keep notes, if they would like, of pertinent material that happens to occur to them. Such conversations can then become a mutual search for understanding the meaning of the experience for both the person and the researcher.

Once again, the nature of the experience and the nature of each person should guide how the researcher proceeds. There cannot be set rules, since we set out believing that individuals are unique and interpret their own reality. They will lead us, with our encouragement. This means, for example, six people may seem sufficient for a particular phase of a study. Also, person A may provide a rich description of the phenomenon in two interviews, while person C wants to have six conversations.

In the section of a research proposal describing the sample, it is usual to say a specific number of people will be interviewed once, with a follow-up to determine accuracy. From the perspective I have suggested, the proposal section would include interviews under a broader existential exploration (as illustrated in Figure 2.1). Within this section, the researcher would indicate the likely number of participants (because the exact number is unknown at the start) and state that the number of interviews will be established from the material and the experience as they unfold.

The location of the interview will depend on the specific context and may be different from individual to individual. It may be best in some situations to set up a mutually agreed-on time, day, or times at a person's home. On the other hand, there may be times when a nearby cafe, where you might even share coffee or tea, would be conducive to a conversation.

Keep in mind that dialogic conversation does not imply a sharing of experiences, but suggests a dialogue where the researcher probes further or asks for meaning, specifically, of another person's experience.

An office may be appropriate if it does not imply a nonexistent relationship (for example, a faculty member's office, if the interviewee is not a student), but many considerations need to be taken into account. Your office, wherever it might be, puts you in a position of power that could influence the tenor of the interview.

So the location, like all the decisions concerning your study, should be reasonable and rational. In this approach, your decisions are not based on rules that exist out of context but on thoughtfulness about the ramifications of your study plan.

Whether to Record or Highlight Interviews and Other Technical Questions

This harkens back to the "ten transcribed interviews" formula that has become somewhat associated with "the way" researchers "do" phenomenology. Persons skilled in transcription make written copies of verbatim (usually tape-recorded) communications. To show the form these interviews may take, I have included an extract from a student's transcribed interview. Another example shows how a letter can be interpreted in the phenomenological mode. A student's practice paper using a literary source provides the final "how to do" example in this chapter. This interesting application of the hermeneutical method demonstrates thematic analysis, which is inherent in the goal of interpretation.

A GIANT LEAP—INTERVIEWS FROM THE PHENOMENOLOGICAL PERSPECTIVE

The method of interpreting texts by going from line to line, or of highlighting them, and interpreting from the part to the whole or from the whole to the part has been accepted as a legitimate form of interpreting interviews, and it is beyond the scope of this text to philosophically question this practice.

Within the scope of the text, however, is my belief that we should not sanctify this process as one of technique *like philosophical conceptual analysis.* We would then come to a written interpretation of meaning requiring a logical linear process. As a result of this technique, I have, for years, witnessed students developing *method-driven* studies rather than phenomenologies. How difficult it is for us in this country to think in ways that are not formula based or theory based. We have been rewarded for assuredness and, as previously mentioned, for knowing. So I become concerned when students take an interview apart line by line, away from the individual, away from life and the landscape, away from the horizon and the background. To compound this problem, students and nurse researchers often want to know if computer software programs are available to do this dismantling. I will be candid; here is where I shudder.

With computers, frequencies of phrases may be picked up, lists may be generated, tables can be composed; but the intonation of a voice, the posture of an individual telling a story, the tears, the laughter, the struggle, the joy, the essential search that identifies this human endeavor will not be there. When I think about the importance of a pause in a conversation and the significance of the sometimes puzzled look exchanged between the person being interviewed and the interviewer, I wonder why researchers have such a desire for technology. Neil Postman (1992), in his book *Technopoly,* comments about some technology:

> *It creates a culture without a moral foundation. It undermines certain mental processes and sound relations that make human life worth living. (p. II)*

And if we are doing research from a phenomenological perspective, it is the human life we are interested in. Qualitative research methods in nursing, as well as in other fields, often began as a reaction to the mechanistic view of the human as a machine. Postman (1992) reminds us that machines vis-à-vis artificial intelligence cannot feel and cannot understand. Programs can be made with appropriate questions, but the machine does not know what the question means or *even that the question has meaning.*

All this is a warning—before we stray too far from the fundamental aim of phenomenology—that the goal is to be more human, to understand the meaning of our humanness, to answer that question: What does it mean to be human? It seems to me that the closer we stay to the human dimensions of our interest, the more it will reflect on the reality of meaning. We cannot achieve such a result from a formula that creates a formalistic analytic (as in mathematics) model for interpretation. For example, a student or researcher doing phenomenology needs to understand the process of transference and the role it plays in understanding meaning in experience. This awareness could never be duplicated by a machine even though the potential for transference surfaces whenever two people are interacting.

When students question whether to record or not, or whether a computer program is available, they do not fully understand what is available to us in our human exchange. There are more pertinent considerations, such as recognizing transference and projection. Nevertheless, this is how recording seems to me. Students and beginning researchers seem to like to work with the interview transcriptions. Many novices have told me they can anticipate eventually not needing to do this, but instead being able to rely on making notes after the interviews. Some researchers have wondered if recording the conversations threatened or in some way restricted their fluency or spontaneity. They report that individuals periodically glance at the recorder, indicating that its presence makes a difference.

With these caveats, what follows are three examples of phenomenological material collected by students who are attempting to implement thematic analysis. The order of these examples illustrates the progression of interpretive phenomenology:

1. Tomas Madayag's (1992) study on caring for AIDS patients demonstrates technique in both the interview and his interpretation of it.
2. Lauren Barlow (1993) demonstrates the discovery of essential themes and also a linguistic transformation of the phenomenon from a letter.

3. Monique Biondolillo (1992) uses this same process and concludes with a linguistic transformation from a literary source.

These examples and others in the text can assist you in understanding how researchers go about finding meaning. A graduate student, Vivian Moore (1993), shared her way of finding meaning from
her interview material (study referred to in Chapters 2 and 3):

*After the interview, I listened to the tape and then I had the tape
transcribed. Next I listened to the tape and checked it against the
transcript. From this, I got a general idea of what the participant
was saying. Listening was very helpful as the tone of voice made it
more personal. A few days later, I read through the transcript
again, trying to get the mother's feelings about the nursing care she
experienced. Alongside the highlighting, I wrote notes on what I
thought was occurring. About a week later, I reread the transcript,
highlighting in different colors to differentiate between nurse's actions, participant's perception of the nurse, and the participant's
feelings. I did this for each participant and then began to group
similar experiences and feelings. I read and reread these to try and
see what the participants were telling me. Similar themes emerged.
I then grouped the similar initial themes. Again, I read the transcripts, highlighting (color coded) to the three groups of initial
themes. The essential themes surfaced. I'm currently writing and
rewriting the homeless mother's experience of receiving nursing
care using the essential and initial themes to guide my writing.*

Example 1

This extract is taken from an interview by Tomas Madayag, who was
studying the experience of caring for AIDS patients. It illustrates an
attempt to interpret the meaning of the dialogue from the patient's
perspective.

The student's thematic analysis appears in the right-hand column.

TM: OK. Thank you very much
    for participating in this study.
    The question I would like to
    pose to you is: What is your

experience of caring for AIDS
patients?

NURSE: Well, Tomas, I've taken
care of AIDS patients primarily in acute care settings, although I have a lot of friends
who have AIDS and so I get
to see AIDS from many different perspectives from some
other nurses would. I think
that the most common en-
counter with an AIDS patient
for me is trying to establish a
relationship with the patient.
From my own perspective,
*AIDS patients suffer a great
deal of aloneness, separateness, separateness from society,* primarily I think, because
of media, of the way AIDS is
presented as a lifestyle disease of gay people, or IV drug
users and *they all tend to
have negative connotations
which separates this as an illness from all the others or
even the patients have a feeling of separateness, of being
very alone. For me as a
nurse, that's one of the openings for me to care.* For me to
address that aloneness. I
think that being gay for me
has really bridged the gap of
aloneness because I know the
experience of being alone, in
being separate from society.
In a sense, when some people

The nurse experiences patients
with AIDS as lonely, separate individuals because of the treatment others give them.

The separateness and loneliness
resulting from the stigma given
to AIDS patients becomes the
impetus for this nurse to care.

know you're gay, they isolate you or treat you differently. *Primarily, most of my experiences with AIDS patients are with gay patients and while they may have made their adjustments to the separateness of being gay, it's now impossible for them; it really is hard for them to make adjustments of this separateness because being gay was an invisible thing. Having AIDS is not invisible.* Everybody knows that in the medical center, or within the facility that treats them, certainly these patients very much sense stigma and aloneness setting them apart from the rest of the patients.

TM: Can you give me an example of that experience?

NURSE: Well, I think that from what patients tell me and from what I see in patients, sometimes how I feel. *When I feel my own mask, gowns, and gloves and stuff we put on to see people, that creates the sense of separateness and aloneness.* I think that patients have responded in this area of aloneness in assessing *the way that people hardly talk to them. They minimize encounters with these kinds of patients;* patients are taken

The nurse experiences the aloneness and separateness of gay patients with AIDS in a dual sense: the self-isolation created by the homosexuality, and the externally imposed isolation caused by others due to fear of AIDS.

The nurse experiences separateness from the patient with AIDS as barrier precautions are applied that extend the distance of nurse from patient.

to X-ray and left on a stretcher, gowned, and masked and all this kind of stuff, and no one bothers to say anything to them except that people rush them to rooms and they do their treatment. *So a lot of my nursing with these people is to show them I am not afraid of physical contact with them,* I am afraid of social contact with them. *It's an attempt to bridge this aloneness, separateness,* and also these people desperately need acceptance and love. They feel very unloved. A lot of the patients express that this is God's retribution or all that Christian crap that some of us had told them and so that I think *the other important call here for nursing is to, or from my experience, is to let them know that these things don't separate them from being human.* And from the need to be loved and cared for and to receive quality medical and nursing care. I think that, that's a very important one. *When I first began teaching with AIDS patients, I had overwhelming fear of contracting HIV. I realize how, today, after many years of doing this, that I*

The nurse attempts to provide care to patients with AIDS in the highest quality possible to undo the isolation and separation enforced by nurses.

The nurse responds to the call of AIDS patients in their need to be reassured of their humanness.

Early experiences with AIDS patients were laden with fear, which eventually disappeared as the lack of knowledge was corrected.

have no more risk from them than from anybody else, getting a lot of other things. But initially I think the . . . this terrible hype about AIDS being a deadly disease does not frighten me as a nurse and making me a little bit more distant from these patients. *Initially than I need have been similarly from my own fear and lack of knowledge.*

The fear of contracting AIDS from patients diminished with experience in the care of patients with AIDS.

TM: Can you share with me that first experience?

NURSE: The first time, well, I can remember, . . . I remember when a friend of mine told me he was HIV positive. My first experience was, I worked for the health department and I was doing alternate site testing and counseling for HIV and a friend of mine showed up for counseling. He had his blood drawn, so I did the counseling and I drew the blood. And *when it cam back positive, I felt as though my relationship with him had changed.* I don't know, I was somewhat afraid of it now, knowing somebody that I knew very close, and good friends with had it. That's my initial reaction of fear of it

When the nurse knows the person has AIDS (through friendship), the nurse experiences a change in that relationship because of fear.

having come home to me. Instead of being someone that I
didn't know or some isolated
patients in some medical center. This was someone that I
knew. So that was my first
thing of fear. *Also being gay,
it's also my greatest fear that
I too could be positive and
that was a scary experience
as a nurse worrying that as
I'm sitting here counseling
people, I'm . . . I'm hearing
myself tell me the same facts
and figures, the same statistics, preventives, and all that
sort. Those are kind of scary
experiences initially; now
they're not scary experiences;
they're more like comforting
experiences to share what I
know about HIV and AIDS;*
now . . . is not a terminal
disease. . . .

The fear of AIDS is brought
about by cognizance that the
nurse can also share the same
mentality as the patients. As the
nurse informs the patient about
AIDS, he also informs himself of
the same.

As the nurse experiences confidence about AIDS, the discom-
fort of telling the patients about
AIDS is overshadowed by the
comfort it may bring the patient. . . .

Example 2

Lauren Barlow (1993) demonstrates the interpretive process in the
following moving piece, taken from a letter. Though lengthy, it provides a very rich description of this tragic experience. Themes that
occur to Lauren are grouped together in thematic statements. It is important to note that the thematic statements are in concrete and not
abstract language. I believe we are still within an affective domain of
meaing. Lauren then does a beautiful and insightful linguistic transformation which includes an interpretation of "what's it like?"

A Letter from a Battered Wife

*I am in my 30s and so is my husband. I have a high school diploma
and am presently attending a local college, trying to obtain the*

*additional education I need. My husband is a college graduate and
a professional in his field. We are both attractive and, for the most
part, respected and well-liked. We have four children and live in a
middle-class home with all the comforts we could possibly want. I
have everything, except life without fear. For most of my married
life I have been periodically beaten by my husband. What do I
mean by "beaten"? I mean that parts of my body have been hit vio-
lently and repeatedly, and that painful bruises, swelling, bleeding
wounds, unconsciousness, and combinations of these things have
resulted. Beating should be distinguished from all other kinds of
physical abuse—including being hit and shoved around. When I
say my husband threatens me with abuse, I do not mean he warns
me that he may lose control. I mean that he shakes a fist against my
face or nose, makes punching-bag jabs at my shoulder, or makes
similar gestures which may quickly turn into a full-fledged beating.
I have had glasses thrown at me. I have been kicked in the abdomen when I was visibly pregnant. I have been kicked off the bed
and hit while lying on the floor—again, while I was pregnant. I
have been whipped, kicked, and thrown, picked up again and
thrown down again. I have been punched and kicked in the head,
chest, face, and abdomen more times than I can count. I have been
slapped for saying something about politics, for having a different
view about religion, for swearing, for crying, for wanting to have
intercourse. I have been threatened when I wouldn't do something
he told me to do. I have been threatened when he's had a bad day
and when he's had a good day. I have been threatened, slapped,
and beaten after stating bitterly that I didn't like what he was doing with another woman. After each beating, my husband has left
the house and remained away for days. Few people have ever seen
my black and blue face or swollen lips because I have always stayed
indoors afterward, feeling ashamed. I was never able to drive following one of those beatings, so I could not get myself to a hospital
for care. I could never have left my young children alone, even if I
could have driven a car. Hysteria inevitably sets in after a beating.
This hysteria—the shaking and crying and mumbling—is not accepted by anyone, so there has never been anyone to call. My husband on a few occasions did phone a day or so later so we could
agree on the excuse I would use for returning to work, the grocery
store, the dentist appointment, and so on. I used the excuses—a car
accident, oral surgery, things like that. Now, the first response to
this story, which I myself think of, will be "Why didn't you seek
help?" I did. Early in our marriage, I went to a clergyman who,*

after a few visits, told me that my husband meant no real harm, that he was just confused and felt insecure. I was encouraged to be more tolerant and understanding. Most important, I was told to forgive him the beatings just as Christ had forgiven me from the cross. I did that, too. Things continued. Next time I turned to a doctor. I was given little pills to relax me and told to take things a little easier. I was just too nervous. I turned to a friend, and when her husband found out, he accused me of either making things up or exaggerating the situation. She was told to stay away from me. She didn't, but she could not longer really help me. Just by believing me, she was made to feel disloyal. I turned to a professional family guidance agency. I was told there that my husband needed help and that I should find a way to control the incidents. I couldn't control the beatings—that was the whole point of my seeking help. At the agency, I found I had to defend myself against the suspicion that I wanted to be hit, that I invited the beatings. Good God! Did the Jews invite themselves to be slaughtered in Germany? I did go to two more doctors. One asked me what I had done to provoke my husband. The other asked if we had made up yet. I called the police one time. They not only did not respond to the call, they called several hours later to ask if things had "settled down." I could have been dead by then! I have nowhere to go if it happens again. No one wants to take in a woman with four children. Even if there were someone kind enough to care, no one wants to become involved in what is commonly referred to as a "domestic situation." Everyone I have gone to for help has somehow wanted to blame me and vindicate my husband. I can see it lying there between their words and at the end of their sentences. The clergyman, the doctor, the counselor, my friend's husband, the police—all of them have found a way to vindicate my husband. No one has to "provoke" a wife-beater. He will strike out when he's ready and for whatever reason he has at the moment. I may be his excuse, but I have never been the reason. I know that I do not want to be hit. I know, too, that I will be beaten again unless I can find a way out for myself and my children. I am terrified for them also. As a married woman, I have no recourse but remaining in the situation which is causing me to be painfully abused. I have suffered physical and emotional battering and spiritual rape because the social structure of my world says I cannot do anything about a man who wants to beat me. . . . But staying with my husband means that my children must be subjected to the emotional battering caused when they see their mother's beaten face or hear her screams in the middle of the night. I know that I have to get out. But when you have nowhere to go, you know that you must go on your own and expect no support. I have to be ready for that. I have to be ready to support myself and the children completely, and still provide a decent environment for them. I pray that I can do that before I am murdered in my own home. I have learned that no one believes me and that I cannot depend upon any outside help. All I have left is the hope that I can get away before it is too late. I have learned also that the doctors, the police, the clergy, and my friends will excuse my husband for distorting my face, but won't forgive me for looking bruised and broken. The greatest tragedy is that I am still praying, and there is not a human person to listen. Being beaten is a terrible thing; it is most terrible of all if you are not equipped to fight back. I recall an occasion when I tried to defend myself and actually tore my husband's shirt. Later, he showed it to a relative as proof that I had done something terribly wrong. The fact that at that moment I had several raised spots on my head hidden by my hair, a swollen lip that was bleeding, and a severely damaged cheek with a blood clot that caused a permanent dimple didn't matter to him. What mattered was that I tore his shirt! That I tore it in self-defense didn't mean anything to him. My situation is so untenable I would guess that one who has not experienced one like it would find it incomprehensible. I find it difficult to believe myself. It must be pointed out that while a husband can beat, slap, or threaten his wife, there are "good days." These days tend to wear away the effects of the beating. They tend to cause the wife to put aside the traumas and look to the good—first, because there is nothing else to do; second, because there is nowhere and no one to turn to; and third, because the defeat is the beating and the hope is that it will not happen again. A loving woman like myself always hopes that it will not happen again. When it does, she simply hopes again, until it becomes obvious after a third beating that there is no hope. That is when she turns outward for help to find an answer. When that help is denied, she either resigns herself to the situation she is in or pulls herself together and starts making plans for a future life that includes only herself and her children. For many, the third beating may be too late. Several of the times I have been abused I have been amazed that I have remained alive. Imagine that I have been thrown to a very hard slate floor several times, kicked in the abdomen, the head, and the chest, and still remained alive! What determines who is lucky and who isn't? I could have been dead a long time ago had I been kicked the wrong way. My baby could have been killed or deformed had I been kicked the wrong way. What saved me? I don't know. I only know that it has happened and that each night I dread the final blow that will kill me and leave my children motherless. I hope I can hang on until I complete my education, get a good job, and become self-sufficient enough to care for my children on my own.

Thematic Statements of letter where asterisks are indicate essential themes:

   1. Men who batter and women who are battered can be well-liked, attractive, successful, educated, and respected by others. (1, 2, 3, 4, 5)*

* 2. The woman experiences feelings that she has everything—except a life without fear. (6, 66)

* 3. The woman experiences painful, violent repeated beatings until battered, bruised, broken, and unconscious. (7, 8, 9, 10, 11, 12, 13, 14, 15, 16, 17, 18)

* 4. The woman experiences repeated psychological abuse, threats, and intimidation. (12, 18, 19, 20)

   5. The woman feels that her husband expresses a loss of control when he strikes out. (11)

   6. The wife experiences bitter feelings that her husband is unfaithful and is threatened if she expresses those feelings to him. (21)

* 7. After the woman is beaten, she often experiences abandonment. (22)

   8. The woman feels ashamed of the physical scars of the abuse and is humiliated when others see them. She feels she must fabricate excuses to explain the scars. (23, 28, 29)

---

* Numbers indicate the sentences where this theme was found. Each sentence in letter is numbered starting with the number one.

* 9. The woman experiences feelings of concern for her children's welfare and worries about their being motherless if she is murdered. (25, 74, 75, 94, 103, 104)

*10. The woman experiences emotional devastation resulting in uncontrolled hysteria after being beaten. She feels her emotional outbursts are not socially acceptable. (26, 27)

11. The woman experiences a lack of adequate help and understanding from those people she reached out to for help—the clergy, doctors, police, family guidance, friends. (32, 33, 34, 35, 36, 37, 38, 39, 40, 41, 43)

12. The woman experiences inability to control her husband's abusive outbursts even though others feel she can. (32, 33, 34, 35, 45, 46)

*13. The woman feels accused that she desired to be beaten and provoked her husband into beating her, that it is her fault. (47, 48, 49, 51, 59, 60, 61, 81, 82, 83, 84, 85)

*14. The woman experienced knowing that she could die at the hand of her husband and only "luck" prevented her from dying. (55, 75, 95, 96, 97, 98, 99, 101, 102, 103)

*15. The woman experienced feelings of helplessness, entrapment, and isolation. (56, 57, 58, 68, 69, 72, 76)

*16. The woman knows that she isn't the cause of the abusive treatment. (62, 63, 64)

17. The woman experiences feelings of being terrified for her children and knows that they suffer emotional abuse hearing and seeing their mother beaten. (66, 67, 70)

18. The woman experiences feelings of dependence and weakness so that she is unable to leave her abusive spouse. (72, 73, 74, 104)

*19. The woman feels that anyone who has not experienced what she has would find the situation incomprehensible. She has a difficult time herself believing that she is actually living this nightmare. (76, 79, 86, 87)

*20. The woman experiences hope that some day she can get out alive and that he will not beat her again. But when she is beaten again, her hope dies. (77, 91, 92)

21. The woman feels that while others forgive and vindicate her husband, they will not forgive her for being visibly scarred. (59, 60, 61, 78)

22. The woman prays and feels that no one listens. (75, 79)

*23. The woman experiences feelings of inadequacy in defending herself. (80)

*24. The woman experiences feelings of persecution from others. (81, 82, 83, 84, 85)

25. The woman experiences good days in her marriage that wear away the effects of the beatings. (88, 90)

26. She feels that she is basically a loving woman. (91)

*27. The woman feels the need to turn to the outside for help when she feels there is no hope. (93)

*28. When the woman experiences denial of help, she either resigns herself or thinks about plans to get out. (94, 104)

*29. The woman experiences feelings of fear and anger that her unborn child could have been harmed by her husband's blows. (14, 15, 100)

*30. The woman feels that before she can leave, she must first attain a certain level of education and employability. Her self-esteem is so low that her ability to support herself and her children is more important than the risk of losing her life each day she stays. (104)

*31. Because she is a "married" woman, she has no choice but to stay in this painful, abusive situation. The social structure allows her to be abused.

Linguistic Transformation: The Essence of the Phenomenon

The life of a woman who is battered *can be a life filled with feelings of fear, pain, hysteria, shame, humiliation, disappointment, helplessness, entrapment, weakness, isolation, persecution, anger, terror, bitterness, inadequacy, dependence, low self-esteem, and emotional devastation. These feelings are the result of the painful and violent physical and psychological abuse she suffers at the hands of her husband. The life-world that she perceives through societal norms, values, and expectations dictates that because she is a "married woman" she is compelled to remain in an abusive rela-tionship while her husband is vindicated for his abusive behavior. Although she repeatedly seeks help, she has learned that no help for her is available. In addition, she is made to feel that she is the cause of her husband's abusive behavior, even though she knows in her heart she is not.*

There are "good" days in her marriage, which at times tend to wear away the effects of the beatings.

Hope is what sustains her: the hope that she can complete an ed-ucation in order to be properly prepared to support herself and her children one day, the hope that there will be no more beatings, and the hope that she will not be killed before the day comes when she is finally able to leave.

Example 3

Another student, Monique Biondolillo (1993), chose a short story en-titled "The Stranger Who Taught Magic," by Arthur Gordon, and demonstrates a thematic analysis approach. Monique followed van Manen's approach to uncovering themes and then wrote a poetic nar-rative analyzing and interpreting each sentence of the story. A few sentences are presented here. A reader who might be interested in the whole story is referred to the book.

From the Story

1. That July morning, I re-member, was like any other, calm and opalescent before the heat of the fierce Geor-gia sun.

Sharing wisdom can occur on an ordinary day.

2. I was 13, sunburned, shaggy-haired, a little aloof, and solitary.

Being 13 affords you the lux-ury to be indifferent and exist as the season deems. To be alone and by the sea at 13 years old allows your mind to be almost a blank slate.

3. In winter I had to put on shoes and go to school like everyone else.

4. But summers I lived by the sea, and my mind was empty, wild and free.

5. On this particular morning, I had tied my rowboat to the pilings of an old dock upriver from our village.

Enjoying yourself is finding serenity in how you choose to spend your time, doing what you like best.

6. There, sometimes, the striped sheepshead lurked in the still, green water.

7. I was crouched, motionless as a stone, when a voice spoke suddenly above my head: "Canst thou draw out leviathan with a hook? or his tongue with a cord with thou lettest down?"

Even at the most serene and calm moments in your quietest solitude, another human can catch you by surprise to elicit a feeling of amazement and wonder.

8. I looked up, startled, into a lean pale face and a pair of the most remarkable eyes I had ever seen.

Sharing of wisdom can be initiated unexpectedly when something extraordinary happens.

9. It wasn't a question of color; I'm not sure, now, what color they were.

The spark that ignited the shared experience of wisdom was more than physical presence; there was an intuiting to see beyond the other human into his soul and find meaning in the physical demeanor.

10. It was a combination of things: warmth, humor, interest, alertness.

There is an interconnectedness between humans, an intensity that arises when sharing wisdom takes place, but initial prejudices must be recognized and placed aside.

11. Intensity—that's the word, I guess—and, underlying it all, a curious kind of mocking sadness.

12. I believe I thought him old.	*Age is not a measure of worth in the sharing of wisdom.*
13. He saw how taken aback I was.	*There is a sense of being startled with the interconnectedness of shared wisdom occurs.*
14. "Sorry," he said.	
15. "It's a bit early in the morning for the Book of Job, isn't it?"	*Shared honesty is as important as shared knowledge.*
16. He nodded at two or three fish in the boat.	
17. "Think you could teach me how to catch those?"	*Recognizing that each of us has something to offer another (despite differences in age) in the form of teaching perpetuates the experience of sharing wisdom.*
18. Ordinarily, I was wary of strangers, but anyone interested in fishing was hardly a stranger.	*When people are able to share their wisdom they find comfort in the individual who is receptive to their truths.*
19. I nodded, and he climbed down into the boat.	*There is a mutual unfolding and acceptance between individuals who wish to explore the sharing of wisdom.*

Monique then goes through the entire story, numbering the sentences and isolating thematic statements:

1. Sharing wisdom can occur on an ordinary day. (1, 5, 6)
2. Age, identity, and stature are not barriers to sharing wisdom. (2, 12, 20, 21, 23, 13, 51)
3. People are more receptive to sharing wisdom if they are alone and have a clear mind. (3, 4)
4. Sharing wisdom may startle you. (7, 8, 13)
5. An individual's eyes may reflect the wisdom in the person's soul. (8, 9)

6. Characteristics of individuals who are capable of sharing wisdom include intensity, warmth, humor, thoughtfulness, courage, and alertness. (10, 11, 42, 59, 116)

7. A reciprocity of teaching and learning is part of the process of sharing wisdom. (16, 17, 22, 27, 47, 52, 53, 58, 63–80, 91, 94, 105, 110, 113)

8. Sharing common interests helps to establish the trusting relationship that is necessary in the sharing of wisdom. (26, 97)

9. The talk shared as wisdom may not be familiar to you. (25)

10. A connectedness in the form of a magnetic attraction can be felt between individuals who are capable of sharing wisdom. (11, 26)

11. Secrets may emerge in the shared wisdom experience. (30)

12. Individuals who share wisdom respect each other. (34, 35, 51)

13. A natural curiosity envelops those who wish to share wisdom, and so they make thoughtful inquiries. (11, 36, 101, 102, 107, 108, 109)

14. There is magic and mystery in an insight and/or truth that can be shared in the form of wisdom. (37, 38, 39)

15. The sharing of wisdom brings to an individual's consciousness something he or she hadn't thought of or had taken for granted. (37, 38, 40, 63–71, 98, 104, 107, 108, 109, 113)

"The Stranger Who Taught Magic"

Phenomenon of interest: The Gift of Shared Wisdom
Phenomenological question: What is the lived experience of sharing wisdom?

Composing Linguistic Transformations

The gift of shared wisdom *can occur on an ordinary day among ordinary people. At times, when individuals have found calm serenity in life, another individual who crosses their path may catch them by surprise and offer the gift of shared wisdom. The individuals involved in the process of shared wisdom find a magnetic connectedness whereby they begin to unfold the magic of shared wisdom. This unlikely friendship may begin with a spark that is ignited when one person can see beyond the other, and with a look into the other's eyes recognize the wisdom in the soul. The relationship between the two begins to blossom when a mutual unfolding of shared trust, honesty, and respect for the other alleviates suspicion and lays the foundation for what is yet to come. Each individual feels the need to make the self accessible for the other so that the gift of shared wisdom becomes an evolutionary process. The sharing of wisdom is presented as an offer for the taking, only if you wish to receive and are willing to listen. The reciprocal teaching and learning of knowledge, insights, truths, and judgments are satisfying to both involved. Individuals may find themselves more susceptible to share wisdom when death is approaching or they are at a crossroads in life. Timing and readiness have everything to do with the sharing of wisdom. Shared wisdom can be seen, heard, and felt in the rhythm and patterns of fellow humans, nature, and/or the universe. It is merely the sharing of an insight that has been taken for granted, but this sharing of wisdom is no easy task; you must want to comprehend the other's truths and may even feel helpless doing so. A natural curiosity begins to develop so that the inquiries and insights shared become part of the process. The ability to let go of your own defined reality helps you to understand the wisdom to be shared; this can be accomplished through the use of examples or whatever means are available to promote the process of shared wisdom. You are able to affirm that the sharing of wisdom has taken place and recognize the impact it has made on your life. When the gift of sharing wisdom comes to a close, there is a loss, a sense of finality, but with that finality comes a constant. The experience of sharing wisdom remains with you as that constant while the details of the truths and insights shared come and go from your consciousness as your life sees fit. The gift of shared wisdom is a transcending of beings.*

The three foregoing examples show various techniques for dealing with interviews or literary pieces. For journal articles, short descriptions are essential; for chapters and books, however, the researcher has a greater opportunity to give a description and interpretation that can capture more meaning. Phenomenological writing often is shortchanged through journal requirements.

A personal example of this is an article that I wrote on anger that was published in an issue of *Health Care for Women International*

(1993). The submitted paper was 25 pages in length and was returned to me three times for shortening. Now the problem is that individuals would be correct in saying the present article lacks the phenomenological perspective, yet it had to be limited for journal requirements.

Concurrent with this book, however, I am working on a text* about women's experiences that will allow for a much fuller elaboration of experiences and meaning from this perspective. The experience of anger then can be described in much greater depth and breadth. Many contributors to that volume have written beautiful descriptions of what it means to be a woman that could never be captured in a 10- or 12-page manuscript.

That might be an advertisement.

* In *Wo.nen's Experience*, NLN (1994).

7

You Fill Up My Senses
Artistic Sources as Material

As we continue to look for ways that bring us closer to the human experience, we come to artistic sources. Long thought of as antimethod, artistic sources can open to us a world long excluded from scientific inquiry.

Photographs, films, and literary sources prompt continued phenomenological thinking when we come upon them. We ask: What is the meaning of this? What appears before us, what is concealed? What possibilities are communicated that further our understanding?

Artistic sources are wondrous connections to the human spirit and the telling of what it means to be human. What is unique to them in contrast to conversations or interviews is what they are able to do because of their relationship to the life-world. The temporal is prolonged, the spatial can be viewed, the corporeality can be many, and relationality is often elaborated upon. A good artistic source brings the life-world to "life" and so enriches our journey in finding meaning.

*T*his chapter discusses photographs, films, and literary sources. Since the proposition has been advanced that phenomenology is not a method but rather a perspective, we can consider Sederberg's (1984) suggestion of "Art as Antimethod." He states:

When left unreduced, art provides a way to gain some understanding of the residuals of meaning *[emphasis added] that fall outside
the compass of social science. (p. 47)*

He goes on to say:

*The most important way in which art may complement social sci-
ence, therefore, is by injecting back some contact with the anoma-
lies, the ambiguities, and the tensions that, at times, impinge on
shared meanings but are excluded by the ordered perspective of social science. (p. 51)*

In the human sciences and nursing, we are open to the meaning
and ambiguity of art because it represents being-in-the-world. Art
challenges us to confront tension, anxiety, and disorder. Unpre-
dictability is not filtered out but presented as part of being. The
meaning of art is often unknown, as illustrated in the forthcoming
discussion of photographs. Yet, we may find phenomenological material in art that represents complementary, or expanded, expressions
of meaning that we can weave into our narratives.

ART AS THE REPRESENTATION OF EXPERIENCE

Artistic works bring us closer to experience in a form of contact
filled with representational richness. Two art forms come to mind.
We may remember the human toll of the Vietnam War, but when we
stand in front of the Vietnam Veterans' Memorial in Washington,
D.C., which is inscribed with the names of each person who died in
that conflict, we are presented with an experience that provokes tension, maybe anger, and/or ambiguity. To see notes attached to names
or flowers pasted there for a loved one moves me to an experiential
level of understanding loss, grief, and hope. I am brought into contact with an experience that I'm not sure I could understand through
other ways of knowing.

The Aids quilt is another example. This art piece is a social, political, and a beautiful way of being-in-the-world that represents an attempt to find meaning in this tragic experience. Because art allows
for transcendence, it may bring us paradoxically closer to the experience and provide a rich source of material for the phenomenologist,

who is always asking, "What does it mean to be human?" Both these works of art call to us, to remember, to know, and to feel. The work speaks to us and we hear it emotively and humanly. We become closer to finding meaning.

PHOTOGRAPHS AS AN ART FORM

Photographs are a special artistic medium. In photographs, the truth about experience is very mysterious.

When I think of the four life-worlds, I am aware of their ever-changing nature, this transitory nature of being, and the choosing that is part of the existential nature of knowing who we are. In research guided by phenomenology, we are always aware of our consciousness and sometimes unexpectedly bring the unconscious or subconscious to conscious knowing.

As we weave a growing understanding of a human experience, photographs often can reveal life-worlds. According to Sontag (1977), photographs are of experience, captured by the camera, and can be the ideal extension of consciousness. When we photograph some "thing," we appropriate meaning and importance to that object.

While our research thus far has been in narrative form, photographs may provide a way for us to visualize the experience. Remember, however, that photographs may distort the reality they portend to represent so we always need to know more. Photographs, as supplemental information, then help us come closer to knowing. Phenomenologically, photographs are critical to our "being-in-the-world" because they attempt to represent reality, whether real or wished for. Wished-for reality is part of experience. So I find difficulty when individuals say, as they often do, "It's just a picture," "It's posed," or "It's arranged for a purpose." These objections to photographs do not exclude them from our experiences because presuppositions underlie all photographs. If, for instance, we arrange a family photograph, we wish to portray a certain image. Even if it is not true, the wish to portray it is.

I frequently ask patients to bring in photographs, but for me to gain understanding, the patients must tell me about the images. These pictures are part of their story with their interpretation and their meaning. However, if something in a photograph stimulates my curiosity, I may ask, as in an interview, for the person to tell me more about it.

It is important to note here that the interpretation and meaning given to these objects is more important to us than "truth" or what might appear to be obvious. In photographs, the four life-worlds are held still for an instant and can only be known about through someone telling a story about them. Again, we see the value of acknowledging the appearance and then asking what is concealed as well.

In a seminar once, I presented the following three photographs (Figures 7.1, 7.2, 7.3) and asked the students for their interpretation. What do the photographs say to you?

These photographs placed in that order produced the following interpretation:

These pictures represent a child growing up and growing through adolescence and then maturing. An interpretation was noted how the young boy in a shirt and tie experienced a teenage phase, typical with rock posters, long hair, eating pizza in bed. Some saw hope by the cross around his neck but then thought that just might be the style of rock stars. However, in the third picture, the boy has finally grown up and despite the somewhat long hair looks "respectable."

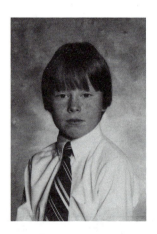

Figure 7.1.

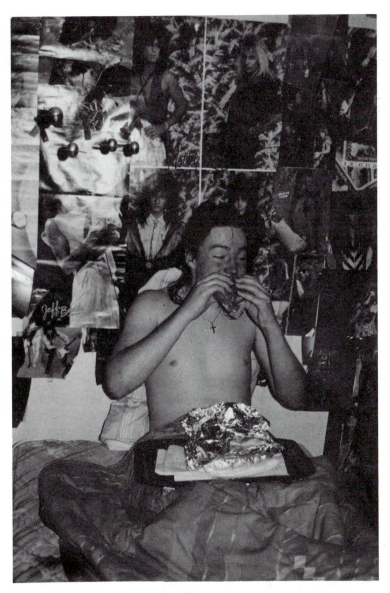

Figure 7.2.

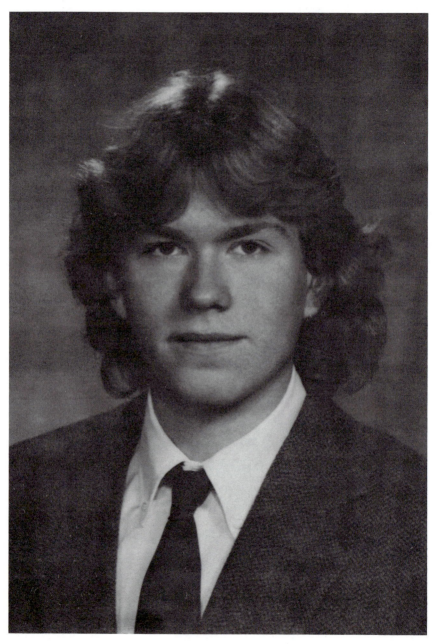

Figure 7.3.

The same photographs grouped differently produced another interpretation:

These are two different children. The youngest one wants to be free but someone, most likely his mother, has made him wear a tie and thus he looks very serious instead of happy. The second child's mother is much more tolerant, and he seems happier. He also seems religious despite all the heavy metal rock star posters above his bed. His hair is long like rock stars, so we think he aspires to this.

And yet another viewer offered this interpretation:

There are two photographs of a child at two different phases of his life. He might have gone to a private or parochial school, hence the formal dress. Physically, he hasn't changed much outside of growing up and his hair apparently now is curly, which can happen.

When shown alone, Figure 7.2 produces an interesting interpretation (the context of the other two photographs apparently hinders seeing this picture as a single visual representation of experience):

This is a teenager whose life looks very topsy-turvy. The posters are all about him with heavy metal rock stars and he seems to want to be one of them. He has long hair, a cross around his neck, and is eating pizza in bed. He has no shirt on. We wonder about his life. Does he work, does he read, does he go to school?

So we know from this exercise that photographs cannot tell us the truth without explanation. They tell us something, and then we attribute meaning to it. Journalists "choose" photographs as a major means of communication, but their photographs often tell stories of sensationalism or sentimentality. As researchers, we need to follow careful guidelines when using photographs as a means to understanding:

- Ask individuals to interpret and explain the meaning of their photographs.
- Use their photographs because, in photographing something, they have already told us they attribute meaning to it.

- For the most part, as a research means, we do not take photographs but use photographs to further our in-depth understanding of an experience.

Of the three pictures, Figure 7.1 shows my son at 6 years, when his first-grade school picture was taken. I had begged him not to wear a white shirt and tie and tried to explain that the attire would not represent him as he usually appeared. I even went as far as using projected peer pressure and told him, "No one else will be dressed like that!"

The picture was supposed to be natural, with children wearing their usual school clothes, but he insisted on the dressy outfit. In addition, Craig was a child who smiled much more often than this portrait would indicate. In general terms, I would never describe him as having been the serious child portrayed in the photograph. I like this picture of him because it demonstrates to me the mystery of being a child. Unless I told you this, the photograph is quite misleading.

Figure 7.2 shows Craig about 8 years later. He has become serious now—about music. His entire room was papered with rock art, and to the extent he was able he lived like a "rock star." I took this picture at 1:00 P.M. on a Saturday, after serving him breakfast in bed, pizza at his request. This definitely was a stage, but it evolved into a love of the arts!

Figure 7.3 is not a picture of Craig, all grown up and supposedly mature, but the senior yearbook photo of his older brother, Dennis. Tie and jacket were required for these pictures. Like many teenagers at that time (1989), Dennis did not own either a tie or jacket. Graduation ceremonies necessitated purchasing those items as well as shoes. The gruffy sneakers he wore to the photo session are out of the camera's view, once again demonstrating the partial truth available in photographs.

Photographs may speak a thousand words, but without interpretation or description by either the photographer or those photographed, we know little about the image. Still, pictures are worth seeking out in a phenomenological study because the image itself brings us closer to the humanness of the experience. Consider a family reunion, where all are gathered within a "posed" picture. Each member of that group could tell you a different version of the dynamics, the appearance, and then what is concealed in the picture.

GAINING UNDERSTANDING THROUGH FILMS

Films are another way of understanding the meaning of being. Like photographs, they too may represent wished-for ways of being or they may be a means of capturing an actual phenomenon in an artistic way. Films, in their portrayals of human experience, can be particularly useful in helping students understand the meaning of being for others. I have asked students to take on a character from a film that I have chosen for its phenomenological promise, and speak the language of that person. In speaking, they come to understand what meaning these representations may have in real-life situations.

The following piece by Susan Manter (1993), is about approaching films phenomenologically:

> *Film can be used as a reflection of the meaning of a given life experience. Coming to know and integrate experience helps to create an openness within individuals.* As we come to know, we realize there is more to know. *The experience itself is the essence, the prereflective time. As soon as we begin reflection, we are aware of what we are doing . . . we become aware of ourselves in time and space. The essence comes from the experienced unaware. Our consciousness, without method, is part of the essence of existence. When watching a film, it is possible to become more than an observer. At times, the viewer can actually feel part of the moment or the experience, and most filmmakers hope for this participation on the part of the audience, whether it is one or many. According to van Manen (1990), some authors represent all of life as a text, but he states that actions and experiences are of a separate nature—not necessarily part of the text we call life. A description of a phenomenon is somewhat separate from the phenomenon itself. The aim is to make the description as much like the original experience as possible. Thereby, others can reflect on the actual experience as it was at the time it occurred. The description must be faithful to the essence. Phenomenology is the faithful recalling of human experience as it is lived. Phenomenological writing is an attempt to interpret the nature of that experience so as to represent and communicate its essence by way of written language. Is the writing true to the lived experience? To truly open our eyes to life and to answer our many questions of "why" to our existence, reflection upon our own essences and those of others is essential. With communication, we are truly part of the world and not just in it.*

Film can do these things. It is not the essence itself even though we may feel completely immersed in it; but it is the representation, the faithful reproduction, of what someone wants to say. It is the communication of ideas, feeling, and experience. It has been written, directed, and acted in by people who hope to truly convey what they mean. It comes out with meaning of its own after being assembled by many people who intend to convey their multiple meanings. It is different from experience itself, even though the desire is to represent experience, because it is done with intent for others, with an awareness of the audience it is intended for. Film is an example of the phenomenological description of experience as is art, poetry, writing, and verbal explanation.

The above is an attempt to orient us to a phenomenological perspective. There are steps to take in exercising the idea of philosophy of phenomenological research, but it is very easy to get sidetracked. Much of our effort is to categorize everything in our lives so as to have life, with our comprehension of it organized and understandable. This helps us to be grounded in our reality so that we do not feel helpless as we move through our experiences on earth. There is a necessity for a certain amount of scholarly input which may include books, charts, graphs, and philosophical orientations. But there exists a real danger in following the scholarly tangent into the horizon and losing the meaning. We become more and more aware of the need for further and further study into an area such as a film or the subject matter we have focused on with a phenomenological question. We probe and question, and interpret, and then proclaim meaning, and then attend conferences to discuss the meaning, and then speak at conferences about the meaning while others sit around looking at us hoping to get the meaning. We leave the meaning behind. It exists in the everyday experience. We ignore the very things we are supposed to be studying . . . living, breathing, experiencing human beings. Meaning cannot be conferred upon or internalized by learning definitions or by listening to or giving speeches. It does not come, in a basic sense, from the words themselves, the text, the instructor, or the philosopher. It comes from the lived experience. It is vital, of utmost importance, to remain strongly oriented in our relationship to our question. We have a response-ability, a natural responsiveness, to be focused. To be focused is to listen and to see without filters or amplifiers. We need to listen to and see the real thing. Our reflection on the "real thing" will bring the deep meaning to light. Van Manen speaks of the real thing as a single case. He refers to the theory of the unique (van Manen, 1990) that begins with a single case, looks for universal qualities, and returns to the single case. The descriptive texts need to oriented, strong, rich, and deep, texts that are focused on the question, attempting to come to understandings that are exclusive of other questions, exploring experiences in all their ramifications, and trying to explore the subject as having more to it than can be superficially grasped. We must be able to meet the text, be with it, encounter, suffer, and consume it, and be consumed by it.

The point of phenomenological investigation is to create in us a more thoughtful and tactful way of relating in and experiencing our world. Phenomenology leads to action. To reflect is to be engaged, engagement reveals meaning, meaning yields awareness, and awareness can strengthen thoughtful action. Everything is always more complex than what we first believe. Questions lead to questions. As each layer is peeled away, greater meaning of life ensues. Living with millions of others on this planet almost mandates a relationship with them. Phenomenology can grow from a research position to a mind-set, a way of living life, an openness to meaning (spatial, temporal, corporeal, and relational). We can take time with the individual that will result in a greater concept of the shape of the whole. This approach takes humans as they are without a previously planned effort to change them (Munhall, 1988). Heidegger (1927) even attempts to come to know the human experience from its very essence—its being . . . the depth of depths, the height of heights.

We may not, in our everyday lives, come to understand meaning in quite that way, but we can be more open in our approach and more thoughtful and tactful in our action. In reflecting on film, we must see the many and varied points of view, remind ourselves that everyone is unique and has a personal history that brought him or her to the time represented in the film, and remain open to change in ourselves as we are receptive to the meanings communicated. Film represents a slice of the pie, not the whole pie; but from it we may come to know the shape, texture, taste, and color of the whole. It is an aid to understanding the whole, real thing. It can't be a synthetic or false representation. But if it is the real piece of pie, we may have to taste it again and again to be sure of its meaning to the whole. Films, books, texts, dialogues, and artwork can be experienced over and over and new nuances may be uncovered each time. We need to really listen, really see, and really attempt to know that which is presented and meaning may ensue.

I think Susan described the use of films and other artistic works very effectively, and now I would like to share with you how her colleagues responded phenomenologically to specific films.

The film *Whose Life Is It, Anyway?* is an excellent film for ethical analysis. In this class, however, we were not interested in an ethical theoretical analysis but in how the experience "was" for an individual. In this particular experience, some students chose the main figure while others chose the doctor's experience.

So it is that in their existential material films offer us a means to understanding. First, here are some responses to the film *Whose Life Is It, Anyway?* The students were to view this film on their own, reflect on a character's "being," and attempt to "get inside" that being in order to understand "what it was like."

Whose Life Is It, Anyway?

The phenomenological question as I perceive it in the film "Whose Life Is It, Anyway?" is, What is the meaning of the experience of being a sculptor who becomes a quadriplegic as the result of a car accident?

I am a sculptor and art professor in Boston, and this was how it was for me. Six months after the accident, I found myself unable to move from the neck down as the spinal cord had been severed. I had my kidneys removed and was on dialysis several times a week. I was unable to feed myself, dress myself, move anything below my neck, stand, sit, or walk. In short, I was a vegetable. My mind had been left intact and was now torturing me.

One time, a student nurse spilled my drink on my clothing and I nearly fell out of bed as she attempted to clean me up. I felt humiliated and sorry for her as well. I asked Dr. Scott if she thought that I would ever walk again. She said, "No." I thanked her for her honesty. I know I will never walk again either. The doctors here want to keep me tranquilized so that I don't become depressed over my condition. I don't want medication; the only thing I have left is my consciousness, and I don't want to lose that. Against my will, Dr. Emerson injected me with Valium. I was outraged! I told him that I didn't want to live; he said I must be depressed and that I would eventually change my mind. I know I won't.

I often dreamt of my beautiful girlfriend who is a dancer, and I thought how I would never use my hands again to sculpt. Although

I felt very sad, I acted angry and told her to leave me and go on with her life. I told her that I could not stand to be reminded of the past whenever I see her. It is so painful. She left.

I told Dr. Scott that I wanted to die. I told her that she thinks her ideas are more important than mine because she is more powerful than I. I see her as a beautiful woman and tell her so.

Mr. Hill, my attorney, is going to help me get discharged. Without care, food, fluids, and dialysis, I would die soon after being discharged. Life is over for me. I can't say the things I want to say or do the things I want to do.

We finally got a hearing before a judge, and I pleaded my case. I know the doctors are all well-meaning people who try to save all the lives they can. But life should be self-supporting. I am not; therefore, I shouldn't live. I tell the judge that the cruelty is that all my choices have been removed. I tell him that I am filled with outrage that those who have no real knowledge of me have the power to condemn me to a life of pain. Just because they can see no blood does not mean there is no pain.

I am so relieved when the judge rules in my favor! At last I can make my own choice! I choose to be left alone to die. I am at peace. My pain will end soon.

Lauren Barlow (1993)

The phenomenological question, as I perceive it, is: What is it like to be Mr. Ken Harrison while being paralyzed from the neck down?

Whose Life Is It, Anyway?

On my God!! Help me. Here I lie, trapped inside Ken Harrison's limp body, but Ken Harrison's representation of conscious reality was left underneath that truck. I have no control, no choices, but this mouth and mind which act as a double-edged sword, a deadly weapon against my useless body and soul.

Who am I? I can no longer express my reality the way I know how to. As an artist, I could let my being speak through my fingers. How am I to do that now? I'm just a talking head. No life, no love, no body. Just here. I'm trapped. Oh, please understand, someone please.

I'm not grateful for my existence now. You all have your nerve! You don't know who I was anyway. I'm just a live corpse to be turned

every two hours. Perhaps, to you, Doc, I'm what makes your percep-
tion of life worth living. Hear me? All I am to you Dr. Emerson is an
objective way to live your *life through* your *work! Go to Hell. Why*
should this place be my only existence now, anyway?

So what if I'm intelligent and have a sense of humor. I don't really
want to live my life without free choice to act out my very being. I
don't exist. Oh please someone, just allow me a choice in my own
self-determination. Most of you mean well, but all of you place your
beloved meaning on my life.

I just wish I could have free choice and some control. Perhaps, if I
was given the choice . . . a choice, that is, to live or die. I would
choose . . . ? Hey, wait a minute, whose life is this, anyway?

From the phenomenological perspective of van Manen (1990), Mr.
Harrison seemed to be lacking unity with his life-world. The four
existentials of lived body, lived space, lived time, and lived relation
to the other in Mr. Harrison's life were in discord due to his paraly-
sis. He could no longer find his being in a new and differentiated
life-world. He preferred to make a choice between life or death
rather than redefine every aspect of his being when succumbing to
the lack of unity in his present existential life-world.

Monique Biondolillo (1993)

The phenomenological question: What is it like to have a patient
who wants to die?

As a doctor, one initially sees the patient as a medical case in the
medical sense. Dr. Scott in the film Whose Life Is It, Anyway?
thought of Mr. Harrison first as a quadriplegic on dialysis needing
steroids and tranquilizers. She is busy listening to his heart making
sure that his vital signs are stable. She experiences him on a very
shallow level first, not really understanding him as a person. At this
point, she really knows very little about him and is reluctant to en-
ter his world. It is his refusal and outrage of taking the Valium that
sets off a spark in her that draws her attention to him. She begins to
experience his humor, his wit, his frustration, in short his common
humanity with her. She is embarrassed and awed by his openness
in complimenting her on her breasts. That interaction draws her
closer to him and she becomes engaged with him in a relationship.
She is forced to shed those layers of medical knowledge and lines of
responsibility and devotes her time in coming to understand who

Mr. Harrison is as a person. She thinks she now understands him and his work and brings to him a piece of artwork that she thinks is his most beautiful work. She is mortified to learn it is not his but Michelangelo's. However, they both marvel at its beauty. His acceptance of her mistake imparts her to accept him and his desire to end his life. She comes to love Mr. Harrison deeply and because of this love comes to accept his decision although his decision brings her pain and sorrow.

Having a patient who wants to die is a journey for a doctor into his or her own soul. A great effort is required to go beyond treating a patient on the medical level to seeing him or her as a unique person. The journey, if allowed to continue, stimulates all the senses that have long been quieted. The journey leads to places never traveled before. It opens secret, dark, unknown doors inside a person's mind. These doors creak with the uncertain, the unforbidden. The journey is not the one planned; that one has been disrupted. It is a difficult journey having little repose, certainly not for the light-hearted. The journey is coming to terms with one's own humanity and mortality as shared with others such as patients. The destination is reached with the acceptance of a person's right to decide to live or die and its consequences.

Vivian Sanchez (1993)

The phenomenological question: What does it mean to be a physician faced with life or death decisions?

I am Dr. Emerson, Chief of Medical Services at this hospital. I have been a physician for eighteen years and I know my job well.

I am confident in my abilities. I like patient work. I can't stand all these speeches I have to make and the meetings I have to attend. I would rather be here on the units working with people. I have a great example to use to answer your question. I have a patient who is thirty-two years old and was in an automobile accident. He suffered a C4 transect, a double nephrectomy, splenectomy, and multiple fractures. All his injuries have healed except for the spinal cord and the mental trauma. He has no movement from the neck down. He has found it impossible to cope with his injuries and wants to be discharged from the hospital to go home. If he does this, he will die because he needs dialysis treatment every other day. It is my sworn duty to preserve life, not end it. To allow this is totally alien to all that I am. This would be condoning suicide. Death is an enemy. That is how I feel about it. I can never get used to it. I fear it. It makes me sick. I feel that everyone should be able to live their allotted 70 years. I look at my patient, and I see an intelligent, wonderful, articulate person. I am truly interested in his welfare. Before the accident, he was a relatively happy person, full of life. For six months after he came here, he never asked about his prognosis. He was joking, nonchalant, laughing. Then finally he asked me if he would ever recover the use of his body. I was wondering when he would ask about it. I told him the truth, and I was gentle in the way I put it. I told him when he was ready. I don't think he could have heard me before. His reaction since then is a result of a need to adjust. He is depressed and suicidal. This is temporary. He needs to give himself time. I can help him through this situation. I am not one to believe that we should quit because things aren't working out exactly like we want them to. He cannot make these judgments. He should not decide whether or not to stay alive because he is depressed right now. It is my job to look at the big picture, and I have seen other people in his situation have very satisfactory lives after they get used to the idea. I feel that I have to protect him from himself in these drastic circumstances. With his mental gymnastics, he is manipulating everyone. I don't think it is right to force me to abandon my values in favor of his. This is against my basic beliefs. My responsibility is to save him, both when he came into the emergency room and now. I know he thinks this is a Catch-22, but let's err on the side of life. To allow him to go home is like executing capital punishment. He would be dead in a week without dialysis . . . two at the most. If I have to, I will use the Mental Hygiene Law and get 2 psychiatrists to agree to commit him to this hospital. People who decide to commit suicide often change their minds at the last minute. I will accept a legal decision, but I still hope for him to change his mind. If I have to choose between life or death for any patient of mine, I will choose life. It is a difficult position to take sometimes and I feel very upset that the patients cannot see the right thing to do; but I will not do what they want against what I know to be right. That's it!

Susan Manter (1993)

The phenomenological question: What is it like to be a quadriplegic?

One day I was a sensitive, creative artist and then suddenly, I became an object to be taken care of. I have lost everything, and everything that was me is gone. I am so angry, but no one will listen to me. If I express my thoughts and feelings, they tell me I am clinically depressed. Then they fill me with drugs so that my mind becomes numb and I cannot feel. I have had my privacy taken from me and am not allowed to keep my dignity.

How do you think you would feel? It is not easy. My most prized possession was my mind. Through my mind I was able to create my art, feel my expressions, and fulfill my dreams. Now I feel as though my mind is going to explode. I have no control over what I do, when I am to do it, and how it will be done. I have all the same thoughts, feelings, and desires, but I am unable to act on them. I have to wait for someone to feed me, dress me, and allow me to defecate. I have no kidney function.

Outside this hospital, I am nothing. So why do they allow me to continue to go on this way? If I was an injured animal they would put me to sleep or shoot me. But, I was once human so they feel it is their obligation to save me. Save me from what? Life? Death . . . myself? This is no way to live. Please just allow me the dignity to choose. I do not want to die for I am already dead. Now, please allow me the choice to decide what is right for me. Treat me like a human. Give me my rights back, and treat me with respect and dignity. Allow me to choose how I will or will not live my life. Honor me as a human.

Robin Petit (1993)

Another film that is most effective and affective is *The Doctor.* From studies of that film, we read more phenomenological material.

The phenomenological question: What's it like to be a doctor who gets sick?

My wife Ann asked me about my examination, "Did they find something in your throat?" I said, "Yes, yes they did; it appears I have a laryngeal tumor." Ann replied "Ok, so we'll beat it." At that moment, I felt the blood rush to my face, I felt my heart race, and my hands became fists. I felt enraged at her expressing that caring crap. She looked so shocked when I yelled through my clinched teeth, "We don't have it, Ann, I have it." I really didn't care that I hurt her, or pushed her away. The only thing I could think of was that I was a crackerjack surgeon who didn't have time to deal with this bullshit. I am the one who gives orders. I am the one always in control. I am a doctor!

I had no idea how it was to feel sick and to have to be a patient in a hospital. You are treated as a mere number on a busy schedule to be dealt with. People without names take away your clothes, doctors waltz in and say, "I'm sorry I'm late," as though the time you have spent waiting just isn't as important as theirs. Oh, and by the way, everyone working in a hospital should drop the I'm sorry part before each sentence because, first, they are not really sorry, and second, at least the conversation could begin with more honesty. Unbelievable duplicate paperwork must be filled out each time you go to a new department. I filled out the same damn paperwork five times in seven days. My experience as a patient was degrading and dehumanizing. It's as though our patient care system is designed to crush people's spirit. It's a wonder anyone gets well! Of course, I'm as much to blame as anyone. I used to instruct my residents not to get emotionally involved with their patients. I believed that in remaining detached and objective I was a better doctor. I would teach my residents to get in, fix it, and get out! I never realized that patients are frightened, embarrassed, and sick. My personal motto was "cut straight," forget the bit about caring—leave that to the shrinks in psychiatry.

It was my friend June who taught me how to live and be caring. She taught me about empathy and understanding. It was through our many talks, while waiting for our radiation treatments, that I came to realize how fragile and sensitive we can become. My patient experience and my relationship with June taught me to stop generalizing and/or categorizing people based on diagnosis. Instead, I came to realize I need to ask "How can I know what this experience means to a person, unless I ask." And then I must be truly willing to listen. June taught me how to be more compassionate and honest. It's amazing to me that it took a young girl dying from cancer to teach me how to be a doctor. It is because of my commitment to the memory of June and to all my patients that I will pass this wisdom on to their new doctors. Today, I can honestly say I am a doctor!

Robin Parker (1993)

The phenomenological question: What is it like to be Dr. McKee?

June, June you showed me the truth. For so long, I had been blind, thinking I was so strong, powerful and invulnerable. I was so independent, feeling like I did not really need anyone—not Ann, not my son, not anyone. I was the great Dr. McKee, famous heart surgeon. And then the tumor in my throat. I could not believe it when I was so coldly told—I was shocked—I felt like dying. No one seemed to understand. I was so alone, still in my world of before, trying to restore my mastery over it. It was you, June, who opened my eyes to the world as it is. You showed me courage, honesty, laughter, and love. You gave me back my own heart; the same heart that had been layered over with anger, fear, and guilt over the things I could not change. You stripped me of my weighted and heavy baggage. So that I could be free. Thank you—I am grateful.

Now, I am whole—I feel alive. I am vulnerable, needing of people. I need Ann and my son—I need my patients. It is through them that I have found meaning and truth. It's sharing life and love. With my patients, I share my own humanity, my own weaknesses, and my own mortality. We are so much like one another. I am grateful to them also for giving me a daily reminder of myself. I thank them. I will use my knowledge and person to treat them as they should be treated, with respect, dignity, and love. Their images are all a reflection of myself. They are a part of me.

Vivian Sanchez (1993)

The phenomenological question: What is it like to be Dr. McKee?

My name is Jack McKee. I'm a cardiopulmonary surgeon. Every day I perform miracles with my hands. I know I'm good at what I do and while I take my job seriously, I also like to have fun while I work. People just take life too seriously, like this patient I saw today for a post-op visit to remove her staples. She says that she has a concern about her husband's feelings toward her scar. She asks if the scar will always be so . . . I stopped her right there. You know people just worry about the most ridiculous things, you'd think she would be happy to be alive. I told her to tell her husband, "I look like a playboy centerfold and I have the staples to prove it." Great line, isn't it?

Well, I've had this cough that everyone keeps reminding me of, so I decided to have someone look at it. A family friend. He checked me out and said I have a red throat, nothing to worry about. Gave me some antibiotics. I guess I feel foolish now; you know, this ego thing. I'm a doctor, you know.

I have a wonderful wife and son. We have a great life, but I do forget things like parents' night like I forgot tonight. Oh well, Ann will forgive me. Well, she can go to her thing and I can go to mine and we will meet later. So busy you know.

Later as we were driving home, I had a coughing spell. I coughed up blood. Ann was hysterical, but I'm sure it was just an irritation; after all, I had it checked out today.

Today's a new day. Making rounds with the residents. They have to learn to control their emotions. I explained to them the lessons of being a doctor. The dangers in feeling too strongly about your patient. The dangers of becoming too involved. Surgery is about judgment. To judge, you have to be detached. The lesson is to cut straight and care less. Someday, they will understand.

I decided to see an ENT, a female, but highly recommended by my partner. Well, she examined me. Not very friendly. Rather cold, you know; I am a doctor and I am a human being. The words came out. "Doctor you have a growth." "A what," I said. "Tumor . . . laryngeoma, I want to biopsy it tomorrow," she replied. Well, you could have knocked me over. I don't know what to say. I went home. I can't believe this is happening to me. I'm scared, but I don't want anyone to know that. It's not doctor-like. Ann is worried, but I don't want her to know what I'm feeling or thinking. I can handle this myself.

Today, I go for my biopsy. Can you believe they want me to fill out all these papers? I'm a doctor! They tried to take me to my room in a wheelchair. There's no reason for that; I can walk, you know! Now there is no private room, and I have to share it with someone. This is just crazy. Then after my biopsy, I get an enema by mistake! It is not easy being the patient.

Dr. Abbott (my ENT) comes in and tells me my biopsy showed a malignancy. I am numb. The big "C." I see my life passing before me. All those things I was going to do, I may never get that chance. Oh God, I'm scared. No, I'll lick this. I talked to my son I don't want him to hear from a friend. I want him to understand. I hope I'm around to see him grow up.

More tests today. More papers to fill out. Getting prepared for radiation treatments. The "system" is getting on my nerves. I just want to get on with this, and get it over with. I'm angry, and I'm going to beat it. I just wish everyone would stop looking at me, talking and whispering like I died. I want to be treated normally. God, I'm scared.

Today, I met June, a patient with a brain tumor, in the radiation crowd. Someone really screwed up on her diagnosis, but I can't say that. She seems a little angry, but I guess I would be, too.

Returned to the office to see patients. I want life to be normal. My partner has a concern I can't perform and maybe I should take some time off. I don't want time off. I don't want time to think or feel.

Today, June was told she is dying. I feel so helpless. I want to make it go away for her. This could be me! I took her to Nevada. She is so afraid and wants to hold on to every passing moment. This is such an emotional roller coaster; happy, and sad, scared, angry, impatient, protecting . . . ! I'm feeling emotions I never knew I had. I want to talk about this but I don't know how. I have kept Ann at a distance, I'm not sure why. I have a friend in June, one who knows how I feel. I need to ask her help. I hate to bother her; after all she is dying. I don't know how to reach out. Ann couldn't understand. June died today!

I must go on! Now they tell me my radiation isn't working; I want to have surgery. I want the Rabbi to do it. He is good and he cares. I trust him. I fired the cold—you know what. Please make this work, this surgery must work. I'm in recovery, the Rabbi comes in; he tells Ann and I that there was no spread to the lymph nodes. Oh, my God, I cried, I can't believe this; I am going to live, I am thankful, what a miracle.

I'm home now. I can't speak but I have a whistle to communicate with. I am so thankful for every day of life.

I spoke for the first time today; I am so happy I am going to be ok, I am going to be well again. I will look at life differently now. I have been given a second chance. I know how it feels to be a patient. I have lived that experience and will remember it when I care for my patients. Everyone should have to be a patient before they can practice medicine.

". . . and now residents, I want to teach you about being a patient. Patients have their own names. They feel frightened, embarrassed, vulnerable, and they feel sick. Most of all, they put their lives in our hands. I could try to explain what that means until I'm blue in the

face, but it wouldn't mean a thing to you . . . it sure never did to me. So, for 72 hours, you will be allocated a disease, you will live that disease . . . all the tests . . . hospital food . . . beds . . . service . . . ."

Sandra Bagaley (1993)

The phenomenological question: What's it like to be a surgeon who becomes sick?

I am Jack McKee, I have life in a tight grip. I am a cardiac surgeon, people put their lives in my hands every day. I know what is best for them. Just get in, fix it, get out. That is what I tell my residents. Don't let your guard down, don't get too emotional.

I found out today I have a malignant tumor in my throat. I want this tumor cut out of my body and out of my life. My doctor says I must have radiation first. I don't have time for this, I am not waiting around like just another patient, I am Dr. Jack McKee, I have been on staff here for years. Doesn't anyone know that, how dare they make me wait, don't they know I save lives every day?

I went a little crazy today in the OR and had to be relieved. I just found out the radiation is not working. Why can't I let my wife get close, why can't I share this fear with her? None of them understand.

I don't trust this doctor, she thinks of her patients as a parotid, a laryngeal, or an adenoid. I am a person, I am lonely and afraid; why can't she see that? I just want to get this tumor out of my life. She tells me she is the doctor and she will let me know when she is available. Why can't she treat me like a person, why is this happening to me? I used to be that kind of doctor, but not any more. Now I know the humiliation of being a patient and eating hospital food and sleeping in hospital beds. I feel so vulnerable. I will never be that kind of doctor again.

I have to have surgery, I am afraid of losing my voice, I am afraid to be a patient; my destiny is in the hands of someone else. I have no control now, I must trust them to do the right thing. My friends and my wife have no idea how I am feeling, they can't understand. Every doctor becomes a patient one day, and then it hits you. I am terrified about this surgery. I know what is truly special is this and now. My friend and fellow patient June taught me that; she is dying of a brain tumor. I go a little bit crazy, but I see my tumor giving me certain freedoms I would never allow myself.

The doctor says my surgery was a success because they got all the cancer, but I can't even speak, and I hate this whistle and chalkboard. I know what it is like to love life now; how can I make my wife understand that I am different now? This terrible disease has changed me, I need my family so much, why don't they understand? I take off my gloves to touch, I can truly touch life now. They put their lives in our hands, now I understand what they mean. Now I understand how to let them all close. I was lonely and with all my defenses, now I let down my arms and they all come to me.

Joanne Massella (1993)

The phenomenological question: What's it like to get sick?

I, Dr. Jack McKee, used to be a very successful surgeon. Now, although I am still a successful surgeon, I am a more sensitive and caring human being. I can now be a better friend—to my wife, my colleagues, and my patients.

I will tell you how this happened. I had a cough for a few months and, reluctantly, had it checked out. My worst fears came true. It turned out to be a malignant tumor on my larynx. The Big C. It is difficult to describe the overwhelming feelings of powerlessness, fear, and despair that are felt when one is diagnosed with cancer. I then underwent radiation therapy, successful in 80% of the cases like mine, which proved, disbearteningly, to be unsuccessful. The next thing I knew, I had to undergo a partial laryngotomy. In the end, I was one of the lucky ones. All the cancer was cut out and I even got my voice back.

How is it that I feel so different? I know now what life is like from the patient's point of view. How very insensitive I as a doctor had been! The feelings that I experienced as a patient I had never really understood in my role as doctor. Feelings of vulnerability, worry, regret, despair, disappointment, pain, humiliation, and fear. Then there were the feelings that come with hope for the future—the complete faith that I put in the doctors treating me (I had no choice), patience to wait for my destiny, and validation that I was important.

June, a fellow cancer patient, became a friend to me. And through her, I learned how to be a real friend. A friend is someone who wants the best for you, who will stand by you, and who will love you even when you're not lovable. A friend is someone who will tell you the truth even if the truth hurts. I am so glad that I realized what a true friend my wife Ann is to me. We are so lucky to have a second chance and are closer friends than ever. By the way, June died. Life is fragile. The rest of us must go on.

I feel that my brush with death was a wake-up call. It allowed me to see myself through new eyes, to see how others saw me, to see what others really needed from me besides my competent operating skills. I can now teach others more completely. Today, I instructed all of my interns to become patients in the hospital for 72 hours. What better way is there for us to understand another than to walk in his/her shoes. Being a more empathetic human being is an important part of being a good doctor.

Lauren Barlow (1993)

As is apparent, films are extraordinary art forms when their content represents a specific experience. Film allows the viewer to step into the lives of those who are experiencing the meaning of some particular entity. In my classes, students who write from a particular character's perspective enlarge the interpretive parts of their study. As suggested by this chapter, researchers studying a particular experience should find it helpful to study art forms that represent the experience. As of yet, for any experience that a student has chosen, we have been able to find at least three films that contribute to our understanding. Since some films about human experience are better than others, selecting a film should be a thoughtful decision.

LITERATURE

In literature, the same potential exists for portrayals of specific experiences that represent humans' "being" in the world. Literature as phenomenological material can be both fiction and nonfiction. From both, we can capture nuances, essences, and interpretations that assist us in our journey for meaning. The meaning of being human is partly found here and there. The "heres" and "theres" are often abundant in the broad, sweeping landscape of literature.

Rorty (1992) states: "Don't look to philosophy for the answers, go to literature." With the phenomenological perspective, we are enriched by both.

As with the discussion on film, I'd like to demonstrate this approach with a few examples. I am going to be rather spontaneous with this and use some books that are here in my study. This is not a classified, categorized library, so I will choose from a mixture of types of literature that have raised my consciousness and have assisted me in comprehending experience:

Example 1: *Obsessive Love* by Dr. Susan Forward (1991)

This book has a pragmatic purpose: to offer crucial help to those millions of people who are driven to "self-defeating, out of control behavior by intense, unfulfilled desire."

Interpretation and description are based on case histories from two decades of the author's practice. This book serves as an example of a short proposal for a study and a meaningful lengthy description of the results. This book can be read in concurrent streams of understanding and would be perhaps read by individuals studying phenomena such as relationships, self-destructive behavior, and obsessions. This book does not claim to be a phenomenologically written book. It seems to me that once a philosopher-scientist studies and understands a phenomenon, instead of "stashing" it in a journal article, he or she could embark on the "authoring" path where sparks of the researcher's own creativity and imagination are delivered to the public.

Example 2: *Family Pictures* by Sue Miller (1990)

This novel exemplifies the "reality" of fiction. When it was used in a class about families, students came to understand family dynamics, different perceptions, the power of family secrets, and roles within families, including the role of illness. Is it fiction when a novel prompts more "phenomenological nods" and insights readily brought to consciousness than a textbook on family theory?

What does this author do but bring us closer to human experience in words thoughtfully and attentively chosen? This novel could be read in a phenomenological study of families, families with an ill child, what denial is about, what a family secret means.

Example 3: *Composing A Life* by Mary Catherine Bateson (1989)

This book also does not claim to be a phenomenological study, yet serves as a wonderful example. This becomes apparent in the way Bateson has interpreted narratives of five women's lives into richly interpreted descriptions of the meaning of experience for living creatively "that reveal grand social truths and peculiar personal graces."

The book is a combination anthology/biography: The method is described in about two pages and is followed by excellent examples of how to write narratives from the material collected. As with Sheehy's book, the Contents here is worth looking at. Recalling the idea of finding themes to guide the organization of material, this quality is evident in the metaphorical and poetic titles of Bateson's chapters:

Chapter	Title
1	Emergent Visions
2	In the Company of Friends
3	From Strength to Strength
4	Opening to the World
5	Partnerships
6	Give and Take
7	Making and Keeping
8	Caretaking
9	Multiple Lives
10	Vicissitudes of Commitment
11	Fits and Starts
12	Enriching the Earth

Read this book for a wonderful prototype. You'll enjoy the content as well, I would imagine.

Example 4: *Girl Interrupted* by Susan Kaysen (1993)

A story of her own experience, Susan Kaysen provides a narrative through poetically named vignettes that describe what it was like to be a psychiatric patient. "Kaysen writes as lucidly about the dark jumble inside her head as she does about the hospital routines, the staff, the patients." The ultimate metaphor of "a parallel universe" and its description and interpretation again receive phenomenological nods of recognition. A literary piece such as this helps us understand the meaning of what we call mental illness, what it is like for a person's life to be interrupted, the experience of being labeled, and the themes of hospitalization. It also provides wonderful examples of paradox and irony as well as tragedy.

Example 5: *When Nietzsche Wept* by Irvin D. Yalom (1992)

Through this author's imagination, fiction brings us closer to understanding the experience of redemption. This excellent literary source helps us understand suicidal despair, mental anguish and suffering, healing, "the talking cure," relationships with duplicity and manipulation, and finally a redemptive friendship. It is wonderful concurrent reading for any phenomenological study concerning the human psyche.

What I am suggesting here is to read widely. Read concurrently or whenever literary works silently transport you into deeper levels of a context of experience created by another who, like you, has a special interest in an experience. These travels, whether they are fiction, fact, or a blend, all contribute to our being connected to the experience. We try to read all we can about this phenomenon, we try to hear all we can, we try to see all we can. We want to understand its meaning. Once we have started a journey to search for meaning, method should be whatever we are doing that facilitates this process.

Example 6: *The Bonfires of the Vanities* by Tom Wolfe (1987)

Is this a novel? It is so close to experience, I have often thought this novel is more a mirror of our society than fiction. The author is reputed to be the foremost chronicler of the way we live in this country. Reading this book would contribute to phenomenological studies about experiences such as ambition, fear, justice, lying, rationalization, ethnic and class meanings, and just about any experience that concerns modernday urban life. "Masters of the

Universe" became a metaphor that was understood conceptually by all who read this novel, and it will always contribute to our understanding of the meaning of ambition run amok.

Example 7: *Women Who Run with the Wolves* by Clarissa Pinkola Estes (1992)

The author in this literary source, categorized as psychology of women, uses "multicultural myths, fairy tales, and stories chosen over 20 years of research that help women reconnect with the instinctual, visionary attributes of the World Women archetype."

This book has captured the imagination of women and is written in a way that could be conceived as phenomenological and political. It is another good example of "what to do with the data" in a phenomenological study. Again, themes give direction to description and interpretation. Any phenomenological study about the lived experiences of women would find rich material in this book.

Poetry, music, and paintings are additional artistic sources for understanding meaning. When you are immersed in your study, be ever attentive to art forms, for in them you will find meaning and additional descriptive pieces that bring you closer to our foremost intention: attempting to find out what it means to be human.

8

Every Step I Take,
Every Move I Make
Thinking Space

Often in the course of your study, you will be surprised at a spontaneous appearance of the experience you are studying. Being wide-awake to the possibility is essential.

In this chapter, the importance of ordinariness and everyday experience is discussed. The grief of friends or families who have lost someone through the tragedy of AIDS begs for interpretation by phenomenologists. Grieving is different when associated with AIDS, and grieving is probably different for many other experiences.

On a lighter side, the entire landscape in mathematics has changed (the report actually used the word landscape*). And lastly, do you see the beauty and otherness of bugs?*

Whatever you are studying, if you are awake to opportunities, the phenomenon will appear over and over.

*T*hroughout your study, you will often be seeing your phenomenon, so to speak, everywhere. That is because your consciousness is directed or raised to the existential life-worlds that make up the experience you are studying. Within this book, my consciousness is directed toward means and ways to help us understand the individual's research approach to the interpretation of phenomenology.

As a matter of fact, whatever occurs in the writing of this book has meaning as being-in-the-world in a demonstrated fashion. I often question in my mind: "What is it like to learn about phenomenology? Is there a way to assist others in understanding phenomenology?" My questions have a specific aim and specific relevance. I hope that we can become more humanly understood and, therefore, would like to see more researchers purposefully aim studies toward that goal. I often incorporate anecdotal material within this book. I do this because I am now connected, attached, and with this book always.

So an anecdote: Chuck and Ray are moving to New Hampshire, as I've mentioned. In just four short days they will, at least, live in another life-world. Chuck tells me it won't be any different—we'll talk on the phone, visit, and so on—but *it will be different.* The temporality, corporeality, spatialty, and relationship of our existential life-worlds will change. They are not moving because I almost killed their dogs. Chuck said he fears I'll move and abandon him. Remember the airport trip. Perception, that is all that matters.

Now when you are writing, try to include similar vignettes that relate to your phenomenon. Another example from my own experience is that my ongoing study on anger has helped me understand my anger at Chuck and Ray's leaving. I've designed a health care plan for myself as a result of gaining the understanding that *anger repressed is transferred to socially acceptable pathology.*
Sometimes.

If I had a patient with this problem, I might explore ways she could express her anger and then transcend it in different ways. I've chosen, and others may choose the same, to utilize distraction, not denial, to deal with my feelings. (A much more serious example follows on grief.) So I've planned to not be alone, visit old friends, throw myself "even more" into my work, and visit Chuck and Ray in six weeks. I'll keep you posted.

ORDINARINESS AND EVERYDAY EXPERIENCE

These two should never be underestimated as critical to research, understanding, and possible substantive descriptions and interpretations. *Most of life is about everyday being,* about how we are in the world as lived-through experience.

If you attempt to understand what grieving is for individuals who have or are related to persons with AIDS, as described in a *U.S. News and World Report* article (June 14, 1993), all the following "everyday" experiences will be demonstrable:

- You will see articles, documentaries, books, art on the subject.
- You can talk with individuals, let them speak of their everyday being-in-the-world experiences.
- At times, you will find yourself reflecting about all this material.
- You may cry, you may find solace.
- Your understanding of the phenomenon may be far greater than ever before.
- You may see how theories on grief need to be revised for specific experiences.
- You might, based on your description and understanding of the phenomenon, suggest ways that health care professionals can better respond to the needs of patients and families.

All of the preceding can apply to any phenomenon, but let us look at specific challenges raised in the previously mentioned article to demonstrate the relevance of phenomenological research. The article is entitled "Grief re-examined: The AIDS epidemic is confounding the normal work of bereavement."

> *AIDS has broken all rules of modern dying, sabotaged all the conventions of mourning. In textbooks, grief is a long journey through stages of denial, darkness, and rage.*

This article doesn't mention the five stages of dying theorized by Kübler-Ross, but I suppose that is what is meant by "rules." I am immediately struck by the phrase "rules of modern dying." The situated context inherent in phenomenological philosophy would make rules of my kind of dying an improbability. There may be many different ways to experience dying, the meaning of which is unique to each person. Nonetheless, an article such as this gives us a description and impetus to rethink, revisit, and reexamine a theory based on assumptions that are apparently not valid in this situation. It is a call to human science researchers to reinterpret this experience based on the everyday. Something critically needs to be "intended" toward by our consciousness. What follows are some examples from the AIDS article that challenge the prevailing paradigm:

- AIDS is a disease that kills primarily the young.
- Families are often cut off from the consolations of home and church.
- Grief is mixed with guilt and shame.
- Grief is felt because of lost chances to "make up" and experience what might be, for instance, a close sibling relationship; it is too late to remedy failed love.
- The possibility is emerging of "perpetual grieving." Since so many are dying, it may be just a matter of days or months before another friend is lost.
- There is a feeling of abandonment from others because of the stigma of the disease.

It comes down to existential values of engagement and participation. Phenomenology as being-in-the-world begs for engagement, not detachment or observation.

Another call for revisiting what we know can be found in the results of the 1992 U.S. census. Human science needs new descriptions and interpretations of how Americans live. The former understandings of families do not adequately account for the majority of the population, if indeed they hold up for many families. So much of what exists as theory needs to be continuously responsive to the existential life-worlds. So while the movement of deconstructionism or revisionist theory may seem new to some of us, theories have always undergone change and revision, as they should. There is a contemporary call to submit all theories and history for reexamination and for confessions of power that have influenced the social and human sciences.

So within this notion of ever-changing theory, here are just a few outcomes of the latest census:

- Only 55% of America's households were headed by married couples in 1992.

- Single-parent families accounted for 1 household in 10 (this troubles me about statistics; in some cultures in the United States, it might be 1 in 3).
- Someone living alone composed 1 household in 4.

Research from a phenomenological perspective needs always to be responsive to describing, understanding, and interpreting such changes. What do they mean about being-in-the-world? What lived experiences of single parenting or living alone do health care professionals need to know, in order to respond in a situated-context appropriate way?

OTHER KINDS OF EVERYDAY EXPERIENCES

A front-page headline of the *New York Times,* June 24, 1993, stated "Ferrests' Last Theorem Has Been Solved," and what a stir it has occasioned. Why do I mention it here? Because even with mathematics, being-in-the-world can be supposedly changed overnight by someone with imagination. A further headline reads "In the world of math—the landscape has changed" (p. A11).

And there is still more. Another headline from the same issue of the *New York Times* sounds phenomenological and existential: "Seeing the Beauty and Otherness of Bugs" (p. B2). Sue Hubbell, in her new book, *Broadsides from the Other Orders: A Book of Bugs,* probably is aware of her existential phenomenological way of being when she states she spent her life "turning away from repetition, uniformity, predictability, safety" and found her delight in "otherness."

CONCLUSIONS ABOUT EVERYDAY EXPERIENCE

As beings, we live through space and time in some degree of awareness. Some people seem to lack awareness, being blank to the ordinary and to everyday experiences. From a phenomenological perspective, this is a tragic waste of consciousness. Most of our lives occur in the ordinary, and not to "see" or visit "meaning" in these moments is perhaps not to live but merely to exist.

The *extraordinary* events of being human are called that because of their infrequent occurrence. But I also believe strongly that we need to study those experiences as well. Tragedies beg for human understanding. Sometimes, and this seems so simple, all that individuals seek during a tragedy is understanding. As health care professionals who listen in a phenomenological way, we can give that understanding.

At our worst, we "tell" others how to get through some experience, based on some theory that may have little relevance at all. In practice and in research, *knowledge screens hearing* if we are not careful.

To apply the word "ordinary" or "extraordinary" implies some normative status. The frequently touted "stop and smell the roses" speaks to us as beings doing research. Capturing what it means to be human is to search for meanings in the everyday life-worlds of people. The situated context helps us to see how what might be ordinary to one person is extraordinary to others. In reality, if we follow an imaginative path to understanding all life experiences, in various situated contexts, we will come closer to the meaning of our lives, other lives, and the otherness of bugs as well!

9

Watching in the Free World
Ethics and Institutional Review Boards as Conscience

This chapter discusses ethical considerations of the phenomenological approach to research as well as institutional review boards as conscience.

The idea that the therapeutic imperative always takes precedence over the research imperative is discussed within the phenomenological perspective.

Considerations that researchers should keep in mind when submitting proposals with a phenomenological perspective to an institutional review board are also discussed.

Protection of individuals has been and always will be of prime importance to human science researchers.

Parts of this chapter are from previously written work by the author and are used here with permission from Sage Publishers.

Munhall, P. "Ethical Considerations in Qualitative Research," *Western Journal of Nursing* 10(2) 150-162, 1988 and "Institutional Review of Qualitative Research Proposals: A Task of No Small Consequence" in *Qualitative Nursing Research: A Contemporary Dialogue,* J. Morse (Ed.), 1989, 1991, p. 258-271. With permission from Sage Publishers.

When doing research from a phenomenological perspective, we need to be attuned to the ethical considerations involving human beings and their telling of experiences. We have already discussed *readiness,* which is a primary ethical consideration.

In the evaluation of an individual's readiness to share an experience, we need to be sensitive and intuitive regarding the individual's psychological state. To avoid possible harm, we must evaluate each person separately. Often, as illustrated in Chapter 5, the researcher bears the responsibility of making a good judgment and considering other dimensions of this process.

This chapter speaks to those considerations and also to the process of institutional review of phenomenological studies.

ETHICS AND THE LIFE WORLD

We in the human sciences seem to be motivated to understand and find meaning in being and that being includes protecting those involved in our research. I like to think that this rigor is founded on a *profound reverence* for human beings and their experiences. As researchers, we are becoming increasingly sophisticated in our qualitative research endeavors and have begun to identify distinct considerations and criteria for viewing the ethical dimensions of the phenomenological approach.

Naturalistic, direct involvement and participation with people necessitate acknowledging the subjective nature and activity of the researchers as the main "tool" of research. Phenomenologically oriented researchers prize this direct involvement, yet contextually must face the canonization of objectivity and detachment by prevailing convention. In contrast, phenomenological researchers face the "nitty gritty," the serendipitous, the passions, the complexity of subjectivity, and attachment to people and their vicissitudes.

In this chapter, I would like to provide one of the stepping stones needed to differentiate criteria that are essential and appropriate for research methods in the human sciences. This discussion will focus on selected ethical considerations while interweaving the themes of ethical means and ends and process consent throughout. Potential role conflict within the investigator is discussed from the perspective of the therapeutic imperative and the research imperative.

UNDERLYING ASSUMPTIONS AND DILEMMAS

In the tradition of phenomenology, I would like to state, or bracket out here, my own beliefs and values and their implications for ethical considerations when doing qualitative nursing research:

1. The therapeutic imperative of the human sciences (advocacy) takes precedence over the research imperative (advancing knowledge) if conflict develops.

2. The human sciences reflect a deontological ethical system (people are not to be treated as means). However, if individuals consent to be part of our research, they have, in essence, joined the research enterprise. Instead of being called subjects or objects, they are now participants.

3. Informed consent is a static, past tense concept. Phenomenological research is an ongoing, dynamic, changing process. Because of unforeseeable events and consequences, a past tense consent is not appropriate. We need to facilitate negotiation and renegotiation to protect our participants' human rights. Therefore, a verblike consent seems necessary and the concept of process consent reflects the ongoing dynamics of phenomenological research.

ETHICAL MEANS AND ENDS

Bellah (1981) sets our stage for ethical dialogue with the premise that all inquiry has normative commitments. Arguing that all social inquiry is linked to ethical reflection, he uses the term "moral sciences" interchangeably with "social sciences." He states: "Social science must consider ends as well as means as objects of rational reflection" (p. 2). Laudan (1977) focuses also on the consequence side of sciences when he states: "Science is essentially a problem-solving activity" (p. 66).

The question to be asked from an ethical perspective then is, toward what goal and for what end? For our purposes here, let us suggest that for the most part human science researchers are very much interested in "problem-solving" or "problem-preventing" research and that our motives are to produce an end that is in some way considered "good." In this way, research assumes a normative commitment, something that "ought" to be. The most apparent example of this is that many of our research endeavors focus on facilitating "health." The search for a means to produce a desired health outcome requires critical ethical reflection.

Other aims we have in addition to or in conjunction with the attainment of health are assisting people to reach their potential, to self-actualize, and to reach their maximum well being. Actually, many of these ends are equivalent to or similes of the concept of health.

Acknowledgment that our aims have normative commitments is critical because we then move on to ways (means) to achieve our decided good. In essence, our aims become prescriptive. An example may serve to illustrate this point.

Ethical Aims

One of the human sciences normative commitments is to help individuals achieve their maximum potential. In this pursuit, we do a phenomenological study of a group of "underachievers" who are not attaining full intellectual potential or physical health potential. The ethical questions that arise include whether the ethical aim is to assist those subjects we study or future generations. What do the underachievers, whom we study, have to gain from our studying them? Further, is it a given that our mission is to help people reach their maximum potential if that help is unrequested?

Although our society has accepted and promoted some goods, we need to reflect upon them. Some may actually be in opposition to others. For example, a "steady state" or some form of "equilibrium" may indeed be in opposition to an achievement ethic. In phenomenological research, knowledge of our participants' aims and normative commitments is an intrinsic component of the research process. We need to reflect on our own and, more important, their normative commitments. This is essential to the understanding of another's perspective.

Ethical Means

In *The Prince,* Machiavelli proclaimed his aim of an independent Italy, free from outside governance, as an end that was readily proclaimed as good. However, his means to that end illustrated moral vacuity. Machiavelli believed that corruption is natural to man. However, by generalizing behavior to all "men," he justified his means in order to obtain an end. Human experimentation is based on the "ends justifying the means" principle.

Changing people's behaviors, often an aim in the human science professions, contrasts sharply with understanding different behaviors and accepting and supporting those differences. Perhaps not all people need or want to reach their maximum potential. Some philosophers, such as Kant, believe humans have a moral obligation to reach their maximum potential. The question then becomes, "Do those in the human sciences have a moral obligation to help others attain a moral obligation?" This is an example of ethical considerations that need in-depth exploration from researchers.

Aims Versus Means

Ethical considerations in qualitative research (and quantitative as well, though they are not spelled out) entail knowing explicitly and implicitly what your ethical means and aims are. Entering and participating with our participants seems a precious experience that calls on us to reflect, know, and critique our ethical means and ends. A negotiated view requires such reflection.

Perhaps the most critical, ethical obligation that phenomenological researchers have is to describe the experiences of others as faithfully as possible. The ethical obligation is to describe and interpret in the most authentic manner the experience that unfolds even if that interpretation is contrary to your aims. Perhaps it might appear wonderful not to strive for maximum achievement of one's potential! Not having to achieve a level of significance to accomplish your aim may be the highest degree of freedom possible when doing research.

THERAPEUTIC VERSUS RESEARCH IMPERATIVE

Ethics is a tangled web of principles where a person can usually see the position of the opposition as having some legitimacy. That is why ethical dilemmas are thorny, at best. In the instance of the therapeutic imperative and the research imperative, the ethical systems of deontology and utilitarianism potentially conflict. The person who is doing research needs to acknowledge what her therapeutic imperative is. Is it deontological, where the individual is not a means to an end but an end as such? Is it advocacy for human beings? Is it based on justice, beneficence, and respect for patients' rights? The researcher also needs to reflect on the research imperative. Is it utilitarian, where people are used as the means to further knowledge? Is the researcher posing possibly uncomfortable conditions for participants? Is the researcher working under a utilitarian posture where the ends may justify the means? With phenomenological research, some conflicts that present dilemmas for researchers are as follows:

Means	Ends
Entry	Departure
Confidence	Disappointment
Elation	Despondency
Commitment	Perceived betrayal
Friendship	Desertion

From a utilitarian perspective, the ends listed here may seem unavoidable in a series of interviews. From the ontological perspective, they are ethically problematic.

Role conflict evolves from behavioral expectations that may differ in the practitioner's therapeutic imperative and in the researcher's imperative. Given the potential for harm, consideration must be given to these dilemmas so as to minimize them or prevent them from occurring. Communication is a vital process, as is a team or joint approach to research. It may be helpful to understand, from a human perspective, that if there is to be a departure, all involved are prepared and the researcher, too, often feels sad. In essence, there is a real "joining" of feelings and understandings.

Doing a series of interviews and conversations about a phenomenon valued by both the researcher and participant forms a relationship. Individuals reveal themselves to the researcher and may feel quite vulnerable. The researcher must be sensitive and act according to all guides of humanistic communication. Although this is not psychotherapy, people often discuss experiences in much the same way they would in a psychotherapy session. And while the researcher is not acting as a psychotherapist, but as a phenomenological researcher, the way of interviewing or responding can be quite similar.

If the subject being studied is sensitive in the eye of the participant, the researchers must always be aware of the individual's psychological and emotional condition. While crying and becoming saddened may be appropriate and can be therapeutic, I think that in such instances we should call within a short time, perhaps later in the day, to ascertain how the participant is doing. At that time, we can confirm our next interview or, if that was to be the last interview, decide whether another interview would be helpful. Strong emotional reactions may be rare, but if for some unforeseen reason the participant does need assistance, you can give a business number where you can be reached and/or you can raise the possibility of a referral to an appropriate person or group. This information should also be part of the consent.

Informed consent has been defined as:

> knowing consent of an individual or his legally authorized representative, so situated as to be able to exercise free power of choice without undue inducement or any element of force, fraud, deceit, duress, or other forms of constraint or coercion. (Annas, Glantz, & Katz, 1977. p. 29)

Typically, informed consents include the title, purpose, and explanation of research and procedures to be followed. Risks and benefits are to be clearly spelled out. A statement that the participant has had the opportunity to ask questions and that the participant is free to withdraw at any time is also included (Field & Morse, 1985). This model of informed consent evolved out of experimental research; some of it is applicable to qualitative research, but more seems needed to resolve some of the aforementioned dilemmas.

PROCESS CONSENT

Because research from a phenomenological perspective is conducted in an ever-changing field, informed consent should be an ongoing process. Over time, consent needs to be renegotiated as unexpected events or consequences occur.

Common sense plays a large part in renegotiating informed consent. If our focus should change, we need to ask participants for permission to change the first agreement. This is important from the perspective of sensitivity to our participants as well. Continually informing and asking permission establishes the needed trust to go on further in an ethical manner.

Secrets

Another area that needs particular ethical consideration in phenomenological interviews or conversations is confidentiality of the exchanges between the researcher and the participants. Both informed and process consent should carefully delineate the data to be included in the study. Role conflict can be generated when the participant wants to tell you a secret or an off-the-record remark. A nurse listens to this and, in fact, knows that a valuable bond has been established. However, the "nurse researcher" and participants will probably be better off if the researcher gently reminds the participant of the purpose of the study and that all communication is supposed to be part of the study (Field & Morse, 1985). If it is possible, as may be the case in a health care facility, the participant can be referred to an appropriate person with any information not relevant to the study. The idea here is to discourage participants from telling secrets unless these secrets can be part of the study. This needs to be done with the utmost care, for secrets are treasures, *but more important, imply promises to keep them.* Most often, these problems can be discussed quite openly with the participants.

Findings and Publication

Anonymity of subjects individually or as a group is often a requisite of qualitative research. However, sometimes individuals and cultures allow themselves to be identified. An understanding about anonymity is part of the informed and process consent. What is often not mentioned or planned for is publication and dissemination of findings. With all research, what the researcher intends to do with the findings needs to be a part of the consent. A longitudinal view from point of

engagement to publication needs to be agreed on with our participants. Having discussions can have quite different consequences than
reading a description of yourself or of your culture or hearing from
someone who has such information. To prevent misunderstandings,
all involved need to agree on the various stages and activities of the
entire study. What will happen to the descriptions? Will they be presented at conferences? Will they be published, and where, and for
what purpose? Our participants need to agree to the dissemination of
findings, from an ethical perspective of deontology, because they are
part of the entire project.

When we have considered the ethical dimensions of our research
and a proposal is completed, we may then have to place the proposal
for review by a human subjects review board or an institutional review board (IRB). This presents many challenges to a researcher's
proposal that contains even the word phenomenology.

THE CHALLENGE

Research from a phenomenological perspective in institutional settings presents different challenges from those of more traditional research methods. The three main challenges in receiving permission
to conduct phenomenological research in institutions are:

1. The IRB's unfamiliarity with the methods, language, and legitimacy of phenomenological research.
2. The structural-functional perspective that pervades most institutions.
3. The conscious or unconscious perception of the similarity of
   phenomenological research methods and investigative journalism.

Although these challenges are interrelated, each one will be addressed separately.

The Unfamiliarity with Phenomenological Research

Most IRBs (and most grant review panels) have members who are unfamiliar with the aims and outcomes of phenomenological research.

Presently, many IRBs are developing guidelines and are uncertain about the role they play in the institution. Their task is complex, and the receipt of a proposal using a method called "phenomenology" may also increase this complexity.

Phenomenological studies aim at understanding a phenomenon by studying the essences of a life experience with thoughtful attention; they search for what it means to be human in the attempt to discover plausible insight. Many members of IRBs are not familiar with such language in a research proposal. They will ask, "What is phenomenology?" or "What is grounded theory?" Though these questions do not spell disaster for proposed qualitative research projects, they do complicate matters because these important questions are asked from the structural-functional perspective of institutions.

The Structural-Functional Approach of Institutions

The structural-functional perspective is often viewed as the sacrosanct way of organizing a bureaucratic institution. Roles are prescribed, functions are distributed, behavior and outcomes are predictable, and all should go well according to fixed rules and procedures. The values in our health care institutions seem removed from or, at best, unrelated to qualitative research aims. For the most part, without our health care institutions, pragmatic goals prevail. There should be an action, an intervention, and a concrete observable task with a measurable outcome. Pragmatism in research is narrowly perceived, for example, as the idea of testing something to solve some problem. That understanding preceding experience or any lived experience can have pragmatic value is not self-evident from the highly structured functional perspective. From such a perspective, the search for meaning appears irrelevant. It is this search for meaning that creates confusion in some minds about the difference between qualitative research and investigative journalism.

Similarity of Phenomenology with Investigative Journalism

All research methods are essentially investigations, but perhaps they are more threatening to individuals when unstructured interviews are part of the research design. Quantitative research designs are by nature specific, the variables are already known, and the researcher searches for relationships between them. On the other hand, discover—the finding out about something otherwise not fully understood—is often the aim of phenomenological research designs.

Within institutions, such studies may be perceived as threatening. Interviewing patients may cause staff to worry about negative information the patient may give such as complaints, the reporting of incidents, and so forth. If there is to be observation, who does not experience some anxiety about the idea of being observed? Fear, then, is an important feeling to consider, and one that cannot be summarily dismissed: What if you do discover some negative findings that reflect poorly on the institution or staff?

These challenges must be addressed in any proposal that goes before an Institutional Review Board. The strategies for meeting these challenges include education and translation, establishing compatible values, and generating trust.

MEETING CHALLENGES

Education and Translation

Becoming sympathetic to the concerns and psychological dynamics of the individuals on institutional review boards is the best place to start. In many cases, these individuals may not understand qualitative research proposals because they may be contrary to the way they think and thus may seem threatening. In addressing these challenges, you should realize that resistance is the normal human response to change. Many qualitative nurse-researchers in institutions have reported that "resistance" was the only response to their research proposal and that they have had to change their proposal and move out of the institution. This situation can change if qualitative nurse-researchers will educate their colleagues who sit on IRBs about the nature and philosophy of qualitative methods.

Most board members are thoroughly familiar with the methods associated with the Western mind-set of objectivity, control, prediction, and so forth. No one needs to explain, ex post facto, correlation, experimental designs, or statistical tests; but phenomenology, as a qualitative research approach, needs explanation. Not only must it be explained, but it must be presented in language that can be understood by individuals familiar with deductive, pragmatic, numerical ideologies.

There is a need to explain in concrete terms the primacy of perception, embodiment, and the philosophical concepts. All these ideas should be clearly stated in language that the reader will understand. For example, in submitting a proposal for a qualitative research project that will examine the needs of patients who have had a mastectomy so that appropriate nursing interventions can be developed, language such as "the lived experience" of having a mastectomy, consciousness, and essences may be used, but they need to be explained. Is this a capitulation, a compromising of our principles? On the contrary, it is the recognition that it can take years to understand these concepts and that there is a limited amount of time and space for explanation in a proposal. So instead of a capitulation, the explanation is actually a pragmatic action for a pragmatic setting. If the institution reflects a structural-functional approach, it is unrealistic to think the IRB review process will not also reflect this perspective.

Compatible Values

In structural-functional bureaucracies, the reality is that the search for meaning, apprehending essential relationships among essences, thematic analysis of cultures, and perceiving another's world are at odds with the predominant problem-task orientation. Helping patients find meaning does not rank high among institutional objectives. So this objective must be stated in the proposal in pragmatic terms, such as "This study will result in improved nursing care or act as the basis for developing nursing intervention." Also, the qualitative method must appear structured, even if there is fluidity and some flexibility in the design. As far as possible, research aims should be compatible with the aims of the institution. The members of the IRB must not see themselves as making an exception by accepting a qualitative research proposal because it appears different from their value orientation. It is best, from any point of view, to *demonstrate the convergence of values* between the institution and the qualitative study by stating how the study's *quest for discovery is laying the groundwork for nursing intervention.*

Generating Trust

Developing trust and alleviating fear and/or anxiety within the institution is critical to a successful qualitative research proposal, and it is also one of the more awkward challenges. This difficulty arises from the perplexing situation in which the staff worry about the researcher having access to potentially damaging information or observing poor nursing care. They wonder what the researcher is going to do with possible negative findings.

This difficulty can be dealt with by pointing out that quantitative researchers in institutions may also witness and be part of the same environmental activities as qualitative researchers, and that the staff themselves are probably aware of any problems that exist. Ideally, ethics committees and quality assurance programs address these problems, yet there is always the possibility that qualitative research may uncover some problems, and consequently, the staff may feel threatened.

The first step in dealing with this problem is to include a category for "unanticipated findings" in the proposal and to carefully spell out what channels the nurse-researcher will use to share such findings. If the members of the IRB understand that it is important to discover findings that indicate problems so they can then be solved, members and staff may be more assured. Again, education is important for achieving this perceptual shift. Traditionally, IRBs are familiar with research that attempts to solve problems. The value of research that may identify problems needing solutions should be stressed, and stressed, and stressed. Indeed, it is critical to identify the right problem before testing solutions.

Sometimes this is difficult to do, such as when patients complain during interviews about poor nursing care. A good qualitative researcher looks at the larger context (before reporting such a result, ethics demands that the lens of the study be widened) and finds there is inadequate staffing. Although the administration may not be happy with that finding, the nurses on the unit will be glad to have such an important need substantiated. At other times, the issue is thornier.

Perhaps the poor nursing care is the result of an incompetent nurse. Although the nurse-researcher cannot be the only one to know of this, he or she is ethically obligated to report these findings through the channels that are established prior to starting the project (see the example in Field & Morse, 1985, pp. 48-49). While this is essentially "whistle-blowing," with its attendant consequences—sometimes good, sometimes bad—this action embodies the belief that "the therapeutic imperative of the human sciences (advocacy) takes precedence over the research imperative (advancing knowledge) if conflict develops."

These problems have greater ramifications for researchers when researching in their home institution, and so if possible, it may be wise to conduct research in another institution. Also, IRBs have members who wish to protect their institution and/or their own reputations. This difficult problem concerning qualitative research proposals should be addressed in positive, helpful terms and fully discussed with staff. They too need to be fully informed about the research project.

Similarities between Qualitative and Quantitative Proposals

There are many similar areas in qualitative and quantitative proposals that concern institutional review boards. More than likely, both types of methods will be using the same form, and the researcher will be asked to address the following areas:

1. Objective of study.
2. Research methodololgy.
3. Characteristics of group(s) involved.
4. Special groups (children of compromised adults).
5. Type of content.
6. Confidentiality of data.
7. Possible risk involved.
8. Nonbeneficial research.

Although there may be other variables, ensuring that individual rights and human dignity are protected needs to be demonstrated and documented. Often, institutional review boards have more elaborated requests than those listed here, and qualitative research proposals are often evaluated on their adherence to traditional scientific method. Scientific legitimacy, then, is being evaluated rather than human subjects' protection. This may not be a problem 10 years from now, but today, proposals come back from IRBs with questions that indicate reluctance to approve the proposal because the board does not understand the method and its concomitant language. As previously suggested, educating members of IRBs about the scientific legitimacy of qualitative studies is an additional task for qualitative nurse-researchers. What follows are some distinguishing characteristics of qualitative research that need to be addressed in IRB proposals.

Departures and Additions for Qualitative Research Proposals

Depending on the institution, a brief overview of the aim and purpose of phenomenological research may precede the proposal or, perhaps, be the introductory paragraph. This does not have to be a highly sophisticated discourse about worldviews and paradigms, with quotes from Husserl, Erasmus, and Speigelberg; rather, it should be a simple paragraph explaining how phenomenology seeks to discover new knowledge, uses narrative descriptions in the findings, involves interviews with individuals, and so forth. Nurse-researchers often get into difficulty by discussing intersubjectively, going "to the things themselves" living the question, and so on. Understandable language is critical.

Objective of the Study.   As previously discussed, the objective of the study should be stated in pragmatic language. Often, researchers state the aim of phenomenological study in existential terms. Remember the setting and take the existential purpose one step further by showing how the study might, for example, improve staff performance or assist the patient in recovery.

This approach is appropriate because it is the phenomenological baseline that enables quantitative researchers to develop hypotheses for nursing intervention, staff performance, and assistance of patients in their recovery. Stress the importance of the study in pragmatic terms.

Research Methodology.   This is perhaps the most important part of the proposal, and it offers the best opportunity for educating members of IRBs. Take the reader through a step-by-step narrative in language that is familiar. This may mean taking a proposal that was written for nursing colleagues of a similar bent and translating it for individuals who may be puzzled by the use of the word "phenomenon." For example, instead of saying "lived experience," just say "experience." In fact, someone once asked me, "What other kind of experience is there?" Perhaps replacing the phrase "ontological commitment" with "it is my belief that" will also be helpful.

Although it may be human to want to impress colleagues with a high level of abstraction, such an approach will probably be counterproductive. In any case, it seems paradoxical when phenomenology is actually very interested in the concrete. No one wants to feel inadequate, so it seems unwise to send out proposals loaded with unfamiliar language. Again, to achieve IRB approval, members must be able to read qualitative research proposals *without a dictionary.*

So phenomenological researchers need to be clear and emphatic about their research approaches. They need to teach about the method and its pragmatic usefulness to nursing sciences in language that will not distract the readers but keep them focused on the substance.

Consent.   There is a debate in the literature as to whether informed consent is necessary when observations and discourse occur during nurses' routine work (Noble, 1985; Oberst, 1985). Interviews have often been exempt from formal informed consent procedures if an individual gives verbal consent. However, I fear we will be on a slippery slope if too many of these exceptions to the written consent process are allowed. Common sense needs to prevail.

Within institutions, phenomenological researchers need to anticipate a request for informed consent. If more than one interview is going to take place, the idea of a process consent seems to exemplify a negotiated view of not only the phenomenon but also the study itself. All consents need to take into consideration the individual's capacity, full disclosure of the research activity, and voluntariness to enter and withdraw freely. An inclusive consent can be found in Field and Morse (1985).

A process consent encourages mutual participation and, perhaps, mutual affirmation for the participants and the researcher. A process consent for phenomenological nursing research should be developed with the research participants' input, ideas, and suggestions and reviewed at specific times if necessary.

It is probably wise to have information about self-disclosed secrets in the process consent. It should be stated that all data obtained will be part of the study. In other words, secrets should be discouraged, as previously discussed, if they cannot be included in the study. It is best to explain to the participants that some secrets pose a dilemma for researchers who are also concerned about the patient's well-being. The question of secrets and patients' confidentiality needs to be planned for and ethical dilemmas need to be considered, before the researcher writes a proposal.

Confidentiality and Anonymity.   The same guarantee of confidentiality of data and anonymity of participants that quantitative researchers give must be made a general principle of qualitative research. This is only a general principle because some institutions allow their identity to be known, especially if the study is going to reflect positively on them. Also, some individuals enjoy being identified in certain kinds of interviews and studies. However, the general principle is to maintain confidentiality and anonymity.

In qualitative research, can we promise confidentiality when we include precise quotations from the transcripts in our publications? The answer is "no," but we can provide anonymity by protecting the identity of the participant. Consequently, individuals and institutions will want assurances that only the researcher(s) will have access to the data and that there will be no identifying evidence, such as names on cassettes, names on computer printouts, and so forth. They will also want information about how and where the data will be stored.

In the section of the proposal, it might be helpful to identify the lines of communication that have been established for reporting findings. Also, information concerning the plans for disseminating the findings (i.e., publication, presentation, and who will receive final reports) should be included and mutually agreed on.

Possible Risks.   Phenomenological research is considered noninvasive, but in a sense, that is a limited perception of the word. While it is true that qualitative researchers do not physically alter the participants with an intervention, there is an invasion of their space and psyche. While this is often therapeutic, it can pose risks if certain precautions are not taken.

It is well substantiated that talking has therapeutic benefits. Patients in institutions, or staff for that matter, often find relief just getting a problem "out of their system" or "off their chest." Nursing intervention often speaks to the provision of opportunities for patients to ventilate their feelings, and interviews provide such an opportunity. Also, attention is usually viewed as a positive experience, and being important enough to study can be viewed positively. That someone's experience is worth studying can have a validating effect.

Are there risks in phenomenological research? One reviewer from an IRB asked about "triggering" an emotional response within the informant. This cannot be lightly dismissed if the experiences under study are highly charged. Because of their education, nurse-researchers are usually able to intervene appropriately and make good assessments about how a patient is responding. It may be normal for a patient to become upset during an interview, and the nurse-researcher must be supportive and manage the interview with good clinical judgment. Arrangements also should be made with the patient's primary caretaker to support the patient after leaving the field. Aamodt (1986) writes:

> In the Human Subject Consent Forms, we had said there were no psychological or social risks. Because communication in response to client feelings is an expected nursing intervention, to ignore such a need could be classified as irresponsible. We planned that interviewers would not be the primary caretaker of the child, and when the situation demanded it, the child and parent were referred to the primary caretaker. (p. 167)

An inaccurate portrayal of participants or situations can also cause harm. A statement of how you intend to ensure accurate descriptions of participants and situations should also be included in this section of the proposal. Validation by the participants is respectful and necessary for authentic representation. The harm/benefit question is succinctly placed in context by Morse (1988):

> Are the risks to the participant any greater than the everyday risk from confiding in a friend? And the "friend" in this context is a registered nurse who is accustomed to handling confidential information, counseling the dying and the distressed, observing and

listening. Yet, suddenly, because the information is obtained under the auspices of "research" (rather than practice), the activities of the nurse may be considered by the IRB as potentially harmful. We must learn to trust our colleagues. (p. 124)

Nonbeneficial Research

This section of the proposal addresses research that is devoid of therapeutic purpose for the participant. Again, the opportunity to verbalize and be appreciated for sharing often does have therapeutic effects. This section should not be problematic, particularly in light of what has previously been discussed.

PRESENTATION TO THE INSTITUTIONAL REVIEW BOARD

When presenting a research proposal to an IRB panel, anticipate as many questions as possible. Consider this to be a wonderful opportunity to discuss your study. Educating IRB members about your research methods and translating them into clear, concrete, pragmatic terms should also be part of the verbal presentation. Know who the board members are and avoid answering questions in a philosophical and existential style. If a member of the clergy is on the board, he or she might understand your answer, but the lawyer, the physician, the two laypeople, the banker, and the accountant might not, so keep your discussion concrete and precise. Remember, the intentions of the IRB are the same as yours: to protect the patient.

In summary, writing clearly, especially philosophical translation, suggesting compatible values between the institution's goals and the research goals, developing trust, and establishing clear lines of communication are important areas to consider when submitting a qualitative research proposal to an institutional review board.

10

Give Meaning a Chance
The Loss of Meaning to Method and the Social Mandate

This chapter discusses the premise that there is "no surer way to kill a piece of research and send it to join the great scrap heap of abandoned projects than Method" (Barthes, 1986, p. 318). Why the continued focus on method when the lifeblood of a study is drained out until it conforms to the predetermined map?

Coming from this is the social mandate of becoming mapless so that we can discover what lies beyond the boundaries. Research from the phenomenological perspective turns and questions the maps, the theories, the taken-for-granted and looks to put meaning into our somnolent world—if meaning could be given a chance.

A major problem for phenomenology as a philosophy is to make sense of it as method in "how" the researcher does "it":

Some people speak of method greedily, demandingly; what they want in work is method; to them it never seems rigorous enough, formal enough. Method becomes a law . . . the invariable fact is

*that a work which constantly proclaims its will-to-method is ulti-
mately sterile: everything has been put into the method, nothing remains for the writing; the researcher insists that his text will be
methodological, but this text never comes: no surer way to kill a
piece of research and send it to join* the great scrap heap of abandoned projects than Method* *(Barthes 1986, p. 318)*

Throughout this text is the thread of some type of method that I
would prefer to call a phenomenological perspective or approach.

In the Chapter 1 section, philosophical ponderings, the word
"method" appears; elsewhere, "how to's" are preponderant. Most
readers are familiar with Gadamer's *Truth and Method* and Morgan's
Beyond Method, which also address considerations concerning methods. In particular, their discussions of assumptions, paradigms, epistemology, and logic are essential to understanding the significance of
method.

THE SEARCH FOR METHOD IN PHENOMENOLOGY

Over the past 7 years, I've labored intensively with an idea of phenomenology as a method. The "form in the service of substance" approach, illustrated in Appendix B, was one way on the path I am
intellectually struggling with. It fits well into the academic quest for
security with rules, procedures, and protocol. Its sequential nature
in some way says that the researcher studying a phenomenon from a
phenomenological perspective proceeds in a way that differs from a
logical positive perspective. Yet it represents a negotiated view.

Absolute reverence for method seems to be a law of science. But
what if the method was derivative rather than prescriptive? What
if every step we took in a study under the rubric of phenomenology was guided by responses to the flow of material? If phenomenological inquiry is "a creative attempt to somehow capture a certain
phenomenon of life in a linguistic description that is both holistic
and analytical, evocative and precise, unique and universal, and
powerful and eloquent" (van Manen, 1984, p. 6), then how can we
do that creatively if we have set the parameters before we gather

* Emphasis added.

the material? In any instances, what we have done (myself included) is follow the same steps of deductive reasoning as our positivist friends to the extent that the proposal usually has as many boundaries and procedures as any other method.

Barthes, I believe, is correct in his assertion. Over the years, nothing has taken the life out of phenomenological inquiry more frequently than the idea of method. I've participated in this methodological quest; I've become lost in it. The proposal outline (Appendix B) is, in some ways, a Jurassic Park version of my own misunderstandings. Yet, it is acceptable because the layout seems logical and rational to some readers. Periodically, its appearance seems to conceal something else: that this just well may be a means to an end.

The loss of meaning to method cannot be overstated or underestimated. Students, colleagues, and myself are caught in this quagmire. The phenomenon that holds our curiosity loses out to hours and years of deliberating method. I sympathize with Feyerabend's frustration with this very problem. I fantasize that one day he threw up his arms in despair and advocated an approach that has been characterized as "anything goes." As discussed in Chapter 1, Morgan (1983) summarizes it as Feyerabend's (1975) anarchy:

> *[He speaks] of a theoretical and methodological anarchism in science on the basis that there is no idea, however ancient and absurd, that is not capable of improving our knowledge. (p. 380)*

Feyerabend's perspective recognizes this potential contradiction between creativity and method. Yet, the seeds are sown so early in the Western world. The rules for method begin with writing your name on the top of the left side of the paper, one inch from the margin, and the date on the same line, on the right side. The *Publication Manual of the American Psychological Association* (APA Manual) is practically a bible in academia. Persons say we need these rules or we would have chaos. But then we do, as in "managed" chaos, and a "scrap heap of abandoned projects."

What *would* happen if we didn't have these methods? Well, for instance, the best-selling book on menopause would not have been written by a journalist (Sheehy, 1991). Not bound by "scientific rules," Sheehy does what comes closest to going "to the things themselves." One activity led to another activity. Sheehy had a topic of personal interest and states:

> *putting on my investigative journalist's hat I explored the state of knowledge on menopause in this country. . . . (p. VIII)*

She goes on:

> *For this book I made a commitment to listen to women, to record their experiences with the Change of Life, hoping their stories will act as a catalyst for honest conversations. (p. vii)*

Could not a nurse have written such a book? As mentioned in the preface, nursing research on menopause is not even cited in this book. We do not know why, but could it be that so much of our research is about method and not meaning? We are so concerned with getting it "right" that, while we are attending to the rules, others are flooding the market with books on health, healing, loss, anger, relationships, mothering, fathering, the new family, women's self-esteem, women's issues, care of the young, the old, the self, and on it goes.

Lest you think I am digressing, my point is that Sheehy's brief Introduction (3½ pages) to *The Silent Passage* has the earmarks of an excellent proposal for research from a phenomenological perspective. Though it is written in the past tense, readers can easily see that this was once a plan that included what could be labeled a "Phenomenological Research Proposal." Thus the proposal takes on the quest for something unknown, a human entity, an experience that directs us further to seek understanding. Because we do not know beforehand, how could we possibly state and design half of our study in the form of "method"? In reality, half of our study is the proposal and the method. In contrast, 3½ pages can include (using Sheehy' book as a model):

Proposal (see Appendix C)

1. Origin of interest in phenomenon.
2. Discovery of a need for study (found "inexcusable" ignorance, little research).

3. Encouragement from public's interest in experience and response to it (article by author generated letters to and conversations with author).
4. Commitment to listen to others.
5. Interviews with women and with individuals from freely crossed disciplines.
6. Phenomenological research as writing.

This is quite different from our current research practices. Future ways of going about doing research from a phenomenological perspective might reflect confidence borne out of reality. Our confidence would eliminate much of what is called the "proposal phases" and that same part in the finished research report. Van Manen (1990) discusses this:

> *A basic assumption would be that the aim of human science research is to create a strong text in a phenomenological sense. And Barthes argues that we are so preoccupied with issues of method that what may really count, the textual practice of writing, is considered a low priority or of little consequence. Almost in a taken-for-granted manner the processes of research and writing remain methodologically separated, since to bring research and writing into a close contact hints at an incestual relation. (p. 23)*

PHENOMENOLOGY AS PHILOSOPHY

Appendix E consists of a chapter from a student's research report, written according to the acceptable form. I am grateful to Robin Parker for allowing me to use her material. This chapter from her thesis gives an excellent background on phenomenology, but it also represents material that at some point may be unnecessary because it will be within our scope of general knowledge. Certainly, we do not see this thorough description in studies from a positivist's perspective because the writer can announce the name of a "method" without 17 pages of description.

The aim of phenomenology is understanding the meaning of being human. We understand the meaning of being human by understanding the meaning specific experiences have for humans. Often, the meaning of research seems to be defined by how a student follows a method; so the demonstration of knowledge of method becomes what is valued, not the gaining of understanding of experience.

But what if the actual method cannot be predicted? What if phenomenology is not a method but a philosophy? What if this philosophy provides a perspective or an approach to research?

Then the researcher would need to understand the philosophy fully, or to an extent that is reasonable (that's better). Indeed, then researchers and faculty guiding students wouldn't be puzzled and frustrated by students who ask how exactly to go about preparing a research proposal.

I can't answer questions about what to "do" when it comes to method when "what" the study is about is usually phenomenon or experience we say we don't understand. Figure 2.1 suggests places to look; Figure 3.1 provides for consciousness of the situated context.

The following questions then become unnecessary:

1. How many interviews should I have?
2. How long should they be?
3. Where should they be?
4. What should I ask?
5. Whose method should I use?
6. Should I extract essences?
7. Should I list themes?
8. Should I interpret the material?

From a phenomenological perspective, these questions would be answered in the current of the ongoing inquiry. The answers would evolve from increased understanding of the material. All our senses are awakened to the appearance or concealment of "some-thing." Even my language fails to capture this process, but the Eastern philosophers with words that represent mindfulness, awareness, conceiving the unconceivable, and limitless consciousness seem to know this better. The metaphor I think of is lying on a raft with currents taking you from one place to another; the pop phrase *go with the flow* captures it for me. Some of my colleagues may flinch at what seems to be such looseness. I defend this position as being far more difficult to bear than having a step-by-step inflexible approach.

The following suggestions will help you achieve more authentic interpretations of experiences:

- To attain a firm grounding in the philosophy of phenomenology, researchers should have at least two semesters of philosophical discourse in specific courses in phenomenology. This could be independent study. Such a requirement is reasonable for its value not only in research but in practice. People can live from this perspective as well as conduct research from it.
- The human sciences literally mean "to know" about humans. Phenomenology is not to be considered a novelty then, but intrinsic to the researcher's practice. It becomes one more thing to learn. In the ideal world, I believe our human science curriculum would be based on the assumptions underpinning phenomenological philosophy. The literature is there, we have come a long way, thus far. Dialogues, exploration, and conversations awaken us to the world that is right before us.
- Appendix G is an outline of a one-semester course where many ideas, thoughts, and works quoted within this text were generated. I believe that course could and should be two courses or more. Just think of all the statistics and research courses students must take to do quantitative research. If they are more interested in the pursuit of this philosopher-scientist path, then I believe we have an ethical obligation to provide courses that will help them achieve this goal.
- Many institutions will not allow students to pursue phenomenological research, or they discourage it for lack of faculty expertise. Perhaps faculty could be encouraged to study this world of ideas by awarding fellowships and grants for that purpose. Students also need to seek institutions that encourage such research, or where they are given the liberty to "try" different ways of coming to know.

Phenomenology—The Struggle for Acceptance

As I write this text, I often wonder about the various possibilities for achieving the kinds of being I dream about. I just experienced being very alone: this is what happened. Writing the preceding suggestions about fellowships and grants, I took a break to read an article I had noticed in the July 13, 1993, issue of *Florida: The Nursing Spectrum* —something about nursing research. Curious, I looked to see what it was about, and this is what I found. After reading 2½ pages about how to read research reports, you could take a test and send it in with seven dollars and by scoring at least 75%, you could earn one contact hour of continuing education. A person has three years, there are 12 multiple-choice questions, and if you should fail (with all the information there within the 2½ pages) you can re-take the test free of charge. I won't comment on this; I suppose it speaks for itself; and perhaps I should feel relieved that qualitative research of any type was not mentioned. If this approach is taken seriously by most, then I am indeed alone. I cannot accept that this is better than nothing. We *can* do better.

Midwest Floods and Qualitative Research *

In 1992, when I wrote an article called "Holding the Mississippi River in Place and Other Implications for Qualitative Research," I never dreamed its content would become relevant to the extent implied by a *New York Times* headline on July 10, 1993: "New Rains in Midwest Bring Threat of Worst Flood in a Century." And the rain and floods continued. On July 11, 1993, the *Miami Herald* reported "Levees straining to contain the Mississippi River: Levees appear ready to burst." The following information, which was the basis for my Mississippi article, partly explains the plight of the people in those areas, and why.

The history of the Atchafalaya River is an account of holding back the natural direction of the Mississippi River. This attempt at controlling nature is what Oliver Houck labeled the third worst effort in the annals of human arrogance. Houck (1987) summed it up as follows:

* Parts of this chapter are from previously written work by the author and is used here with permission from Mosby-Year Book, Inc. Munhall, P. "Holding the Mississippi River in Place and Other Implications for Qualitative Research," *Nursing Outlook,* Nov./Dec., 1992, Vol. 40, No. 6, 257–262.

The greatest arrogance was the stealing of the sun, the second greatest arrogance is running rivers backwards, and third greatest arrogance is trying to hold the Mississippi in place.

The Mississippi River is emptying and filling into the Atchafalaya River. Could technology prevent this? The Army Corps of Engineers thought so, and one of their officials said, "We can't let that happen. We are charged by Congress not to let that happen."

In 1973, the worst flood (before 1993) occurred, and geologists and hydrologic engineers believed that this project was doomed. Rachel Kazmann said:

Nobody knows where the 100-year flood is. Perspective should be a minimum of 100 years. . . . A 50-year prediction is not reliable. The data have lost their pristine character—The Corps of Engineers—they're scared as hell. They don't know what's going to happen. This is planned chaos. The more planning they do, the more chaotic it is. Nobody knows exactly where it's going to end.

Postman (1992) would call this the surrender of culture to technology. It is a state of mind that deifies technology. This new social order proceeds under philosophical assumptions that idealize technology without reflecting on consequences or meanings. Bronowski (1965) states, "This is the paradox of imagination in science, that it has for its aim the impoverishment of imagination."

So while some people in the human sciences are concerned with meaning and imagination, I must confess to what I experience as tolerance (and sometimes not even that), and I do feel alone. Other individuals pursuing the "I'd rather have meaning" approach to research share with me similar uphill, lonely struggles. Why should this be so, when the metaphor of the river is happening in health care today?

THE SOCIAL MANDATE TO FIND MEANING

I understand the politics of meaning, and I recognize that they differ from the politics of "science" (Sederberg, 1984). This section will elaborate on this difference in view, and call on us as researchers to demonstrate the usefulness of our findings. We may be philosopher-scientists, but we cannot afford to be armchair philosophers.

So the saga of the Mississippi continues, as does the advance of science. The dikes, the levees, the outbanks, the billions of dollars are all set in motion. Once these are in place, alternatives are not even searched for. Imagination has been replaced by technological knowledge, and that is how we plug the hole in the dike.

The parallel with the health care system's problems and approach is evident. It begs for alternatives, for acknowledgment of new perspectives, and for the understanding of meaning to assume priority in decision making. I and others worry because, as in the Mississippi project, once the traditional view is set in motion, it proceeds without anyone reflecting on its consequences or its meanings.

This discussion, by means of metaphor, aims at the notion of freedom in nature and, by contrast, freedom in knowledge development. The enlargement of our knowledge base is similar to tributaries that flow from rivers, as depicted in Figure 10.1.

Seemingly flowing upstream, Figure 10.1 reemphasizes the phenomenological perspective in nursing knowledge development. This perspective has many adherents; however, I argue for some strategies that might move this perspective more into the mainstream. This is critical because, as human science researchers, we

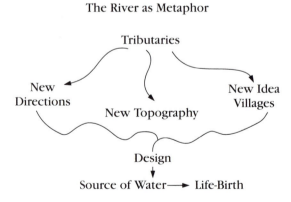

Figure 10.1. River as Metaphor.

have an ethical imperative to respond to the society we serve—a society that has made *Final Exit* a best seller and the Patient Self-Determination Act a law. Spending a third of our health dollar to keep people alive in their last month of life, when they often wish to die peacefully and in comfort, should prompt the human science researcher to fulfill what it is that society wants. Because the ultimate aim of phenomenological research is "the fulfillment of our human nature," it is (as has been stated elsewhere) compatible with human science goals and values.

The Health Care Financing Administration reported in 1990 that the United States spent $660 billion on health care and further projected that the cost of health care will rise to $1.8 trillion by the year 2000.

We must ask the *phenomenological questions* because we do indeed have our being in a lived time and lived space of limited resources. Literally to spend trillions *without reflection as to meaning* is utter foolishness, if not insanity.

While science seems intent with the notion of keeping people alive with technology that costs billions, human beings are begging, not to be kept alive in ways that violate their dignity but to be permitted a peaceful death, within the scope of being human. There is meaning in the experience of dying and, like the engineers who build the levees and dikes, oftentimes health care professionals, with good intentions, don't seem to revere the forces of nature. In the scope of living, of being, is also the eventual natural ending, as we know it: nonbeing. Nature will sometimes have its way.

Now I know that *researchers* using a *phenomenological perspective* are hardly the researchers usually thought of as *reducing the health care budget,* but I say unequivocally that this direction has much promise in doing just that. It may not be its purpose, but the potential for understanding the meaning of what individuals do and why they do it is critical knowledge.

Though our intent is not necessarily to change people, there is an intent to understand experiences in ways that are interpreted by the individual rather than our superimposed interpretation. With that, we might direct our education programs for prevention, question our intervention, and perhaps give to patients what they want and need from their perspective, rather than ours. At the very least, it's a different possibility of being with another that more closely resembles their reality.

With phenomenology's emphasis on the experiences of human beings, many of these researchers are begging the question of where the humanity in health care is. While we applaud the advances of technology and interventions, their ethical use—where and how and particularly choice—must be brought to the fore. We must scrutinize technology, not when the embryos are frozen but before they are frozen.

We also need to design our qualitative research proposals, projects, and findings creatively, in ways that explicitly address situated contexts (for instance, the U.S. Department of Health and Human Service's Health Promotion and Disease Prevention objectives of "Healthy People 2000"). In other words, we begin to fit.

Many qualitative nurse researchers have opted not to pursue funding. I believe such an action has profound meaning because funding is equated with worth. It is said that many of our colleagues are still not convinced that the new rivers are essential for new life. They are not convinced that our ways of coming to know about individuals living as they do can have far-reaching implications in the understanding of why people become sick in the first place. We have not adequately convinced our colleagues that our methods of inquiry often lead us to ask the right research questions for other studies, such as those the Institute for Nursing wishes to pursue. It seems that qualitative nurse researchers are viewed as somehow soft, kind, caring, well-meaning people who perhaps can be nice to patients, while the assessment, management, and measurement people will take care of the real world. We need to dispense with this myth that qualitative research is not powerful, critical to our practice, and an extremely complex activity.

Qualitative research could give direction to practice that would prevent some of the diseases that billions of dollars will be spent on. But this may not occur by doing qualitative research that leads to a one-sentence definition or a structural descriptive statement. The findings we discover should be either descriptive or interpretive in expanse to give us the direction and full-bodied knowing about something that has implications for further research or direct practice implications.

And those direct practice implications are not just limited to say-ing we have some understanding of a phenomenon right now but also to suggesting what might we do based on that understanding. Human science researchers who research from the phenomenologi-cal and qualitative perspectives have the potential to discover what precedes specific lived experiences, what can prevent them (if that should promote quality of life), or what constitutes lived experiences so we can interpret what people need to tolerate, manage, or even enhance them.

While the research agendas being funded speak to putting fires out, nurses of a qualitative leaning know we can prevent fires if we come to understand how they get started in the first place. And if there is a fire, we can learn what people need to live through the experience as human beings and, perhaps, to prevent further injury.

I sometimes sense a lingering apology on the part of researchers for pursuing this form of inquiry. As a phenomenologically based researcher, I can understand that. Perhaps because we want to em-body our embodiment in a phenomenological way of being, we have been too "nice," too understanding. I suggest that our agenda must include the message that the genesis and birth of new discov-eries may require pursuing new tributaries or streams of thought about qualitative research methods. Here are some streams of thought that we might discuss to move ahead, thoughts to ponder as we make our journey.

Pragmatic Pursuits

We need to speak the language of the dominant culture. It matches the lived world and values of the people we study. Phenomenological research needs pragmatic purpose. Why study the lived experience of anger as expressed by women? Because in my research of specific clinical experience I kept hearing recurring psychosomatic themes that had to do with hypertension, depression, cancer, eating disor-ders, obesity, interpersonal struggles, and social and personal self-destructiveness (Munhall, 1993).

In another way of speaking, the research led to a discovery that has the potential to prevent some conditions and symptoms by instituting treatment or intervention at the level of a repressed emotion rather than at the symptom level.

Preventive Pursuits

Closely aligned with the preceding, almost every symptom or behavior is a manifestation of something else, an unmet need, a repressed feeling. Phenomenological research leads to such findings. Bulimia and anorexia are not "eating disorders." The field of psychoneuroimmunology needs phenomenological studies to enable such understandings. Qualitative studies often get under the surface or behind the mask of symptoms and illness.

For instance, we know that life-style changes would prevent much disease. *But we do not really understand life-styles.* Perhaps we have not studied the "meanings" these life-styles hold for individuals. Until then, we will continue to treat life-style outcomes instead of basing our knowledge on understanding of meaning from being-in-the-world.

Interventions and Outcome Pursuits

Purists may not want to travel along this stream, but if qualitative researchers are to gain acknowledgment, they must give direction for practice from their phenomenological research. It may well be that our research need not purposely be hypothesis generating; nonetheless, every good phenomenological study should give direction for practice, and that direction is often not sufficiently discussed. We must say what our research is talking to us about. Somewhere the idea that qualitative research is not about interventions was misconstrued. It is not about testing interventions, but if phenomenological description leads to a different way of responding to a phenomenon, then that should be clearly stated. When people tell us what it is like to experience a life event, we have material with which to design specific plans for nursing care.

Understanding is perhaps one of the most important gifts one human being can give to another. If we learn not only with our minds but with our spirits, the meanings of experience, we might better be able to say, "I understand." People reach out for this, bemoan that no one understands, beg for understanding in their choices. Many practitioners in the mental health care field believe it is understanding or feeling understood that cures the person.

Isn't that what we all wish for . . . to be understood?

Stand and Deliver *Pursuit*

The film *Stand and Deliver* demonstrates that, despite apparently insurmountable obstacles, people can succeed through perseverance, conviction in the value of their work, and the ability to stand up for those beliefs. This is the challenge for researchers exploring the transiency of our prevailing myths and theories and giving life to the reconstruction of a new way of being with others. Not because we are nice (though we may be) but because we are human science researchers.

We must be a voice that is heard. We must acknowledge the present pragmatism and show how our research gives direction to practice and further research.

Our publications should be monographs or books—the average 15-page limit of articles perhaps has impeded others' understanding of our worth. It might also be helpful if articles for publication could take on a more narrative form, with references that direct readers to further elaboration of the research.

Our nursing knowledge base must include the human experience. Becoming oriented to a world of meaning will enlighten and give direction to our practice. The unexamined taken-for-granted approach misses the essential dimensions of being that may actualize the possibilities of new ideas, new directions, new designs, new life, and birth.

11

Tugging at a Piece of My Heart
One P and Ten R's for Evaluation

The purpose of this chapter is to give researchers ways and means of evaluating their phenomenological studies.

The "nod" and resonancy are affective responses. The affective responses are perhaps the most authentic means of knowing whether your study "rings" and "raises" consciousness. Rilke's (1957) Possibility of Being is an inspiration when thinking about "how do I know this is so?" His work tugs at a piece of my heart.

*M*y criteria for evaluating a phenomenological study reflect the original intent of this book, which is in part not to distance the reader or researcher. I have, therefore, tried to make these criteria less abstract and more concrete. In doing so, I do not believe I have sacrificed rigor but rather have developed criteria that are closer to our everyday language and our being with these studies.

I confess to the use of a form of alliteration, with the simple premise that it is easier to "R"ecall another word starting with "R."

ESTABLISHING THE DETERMINANTS OF RIGOR

During a recent summer workshop on the phenomenological perspective in human science, many participants were concerned about reliability and validity. They talked of Guba and Lincoln (1981) using the following criteria to determine methodological rigor of qualitative scientific inquiry: truth value, applicability, consistency, and neutrality. Whether a description of experience is credible to the person who has had the experience is a primary consideration. The second test of validity is the applicability of qualitative research, which is evaluated by "fit" of data into contexts outside the study situation. The consistent results generated by multiple methods of data collection and existential investigation of artistic sources contribute to validity. Findings can be consistent throughout data collection during interviews and should be confirmed with participants as the study is completed. Preliminary findings should be shared and should resonate with the participants.

In the following description of methodological rigor by Maribel Mezquita (1993), she refers to the criteria developed by Burns (1988) for evaluating the rigor of her own phenomenological research:

Methodological Rigor

Criteria for evaluating the qualitative research are presented by Burns (1988). The researcher will ensure adherence to such standards throughout the study. They are the following: (a) descriptive vividness; (b) methodological congruence; (c) analytical preciseness; (d) theoretical connectedness; and (e) heuristic relevance. Burns addresses potential threats to these standards.

In complying with descriptive vividness, the description of the site, the participants, and the researcher's decisions during the study will be clearly presented. The aim will be to inspire the reader to personally experience the event. In eluding threats to descriptive vividness, high level of self-awareness will be maintained and ample observational skills will be incorporated. The use of a transcriptionist will ensure accuracy of the written descriptions.

It is important that the researcher relate to the reader the methodological approach that was used, in order to comply with requirements for methodological congruence. Burns (1988) describes four dimensions within methodological excellence. They are as follows: "rigor in documentation; procedural rigor; ethical rigor; and auditability" (p. 48).

In complying with rigor in documentation, all the elements of the study should be presented in the study. Several of these such as: the phenomenon, purpose, research question, justification for the study, sampling and setting, ethical implications, and general steps have been explained. Others will be displayed as the study advances.

To certify that procedural rigor is maintained, I will clarify the steps and attest that data are accurately collected, recorded, and displayed. The researcher will practice "bracketing" in order to discover the experiences of participants. This will prevent the introduction of biases, from allowing assumptions or preconceived judgments to influence the process of data gathering and analysis. Since the researcher is the instrument for the data collection, the art of bracketing will ensure reliability during the data analysis. I will be working under the supervision of a thesis committee, who will review all the steps of the study to set off any threats under procedural rigor. The interviews will not be timed in order to allow participants plentiful time for reflections and expressions. Sufficient data will be collected and all data collected from descriptions will be analyzed. Ethical rigor will be guaranteed by obtaining written process consent from the participants, prior to collecting data. Such consent acknowledges and protects the individuals' rights throughout the study (Burns, 1988). Auditability will be conferred by providing rationale for the decisions involved in the evolution of the data into the theoretical scheme. This will help other researchers to arrive at similar conclusions by following the decision trail of the investigator. To avert any threats to auditability, I will explain how the themes are developed in the study.

According to Burns (1988), it is essential that the author make a profound effort "to identify and to record the decision-making processes through which transformations were made" (p. 50). This criterion is required to meet analytical preciseness. This report will incorporate rich excerpts from the transcripts as to allow the reader in following with the course of analysis and the evolvement of themes. I will indicate if any data were rejected. The schema or themes will be checked with the original data for proper fittingness and representation. This process will be guided by experienced researchers in phenomenology.

"Theoretical connectedness requires that the theoretical schema developed from the study be clearly expressed, logically consistent, reflective of the data, and compatible with the knowledge base of

nursing" (Burns 1988, p. 50). In complying with theoretical connect-edness, I will ensure that the language of the participants will be used in the emerging themes. Then, these themes will be compared with other existing theories and available nursing research.

Finally, the results of the study need to provide the reader with heuristic relevance. According to Burns (1988) "there are three di-mensions of heuristic relevance: intuitive recognition; relationship to existing body of knowledge; and applicability" (p. 51). Intuitive recognition will be attempted by clearly describing the lived experi-ence in light of its relevance to nursing practice. The finding of the study will be compared to the existing body of knowledge in nursing. Applicability will be achieved by discussing the relevance of these findings in relation to nursing practice and theory development.

ANOTHER PERCEPTION OF
METHODOLOGICAL CRITERIA

Because phenomenological research is based on different philosoph-ical assumptions, I have attempted to develop criteria for evaluation of phenomenological research based on some of the assumptions in this book. Such criteria seem, for me, to better address the everyday concerns about phenomenology consistent with its aims. So what do we do about the rigor of our endeavor to understand the meaning of being human, a rather lofty yet almost attainable goal? First, we need to accept our limitations because it is a big, lofty, philosophical aim. Second, we must realize that we are pursuing understanding of meaning by studying the experience of beings in situated contexts so that we may return to the larger question.

Rigor or merit are as critical to a phenomenologist as they are to an experimental researcher. If the phenomenological baseline has not been meticulously explored and described, then what follows, as in an experiment, will not be congruent with the connected underpin-nings. It simply will not hold up.

Research from a phenomenological perspective should give direc-tion to practice or further research. So the rigor and merit are critical. The criteria for evaluating the phenomenological approach in re-search have often been general and applied to other qualitative meth-ods as well. During the summer seminar referred to earlier, a more specific way to evaluate this research seemed to evolve. You will not be wrong to choose other criteria, but I present the following for your consideration.

One P, Ten R's

Evaluating research from a phenomenological perspective for rigor and merit involves, first of all, assessing the affirmation—the "phenomenological nod"—of your participants.

The Phenomenological Nod.   This occurs when people reading or hearing your presentation nod in agreement. The first phenomenological nod you wish to have is from those participants who spoke with you. It is critical that you as a researcher return to your participants with your study. The participants are the only ones who can answer the question as to whether you have captured their telling of the experience and the meaning the experience held for them. The description and interpretation may not represent *fully* the meaning of the experience for each participant since the descriptions will be different. Often, participants see themselves somewhere in your writings but not necessarily in the entire piece of writing. That is why, in writing, you may find yourself telling a story of a few individuals and then writing the word "however." "However," other participants seemed to interpret a different meaning concerning this experience. This is fine, represents different situated contexts, tells us about our differences, and the variation of attached meanings. In contrast to quantitative goals, the idea of a mean, median, or mode is not useful. In fact, if we write the words "most participants . . ." this phrase does not necessarily mean that we have found a norm in the way we would be seeking norms in other kinds of research. If it happens, fine; if it doesn't, fine. If there is one lived experience with many different interpretive meanings, that itself becomes a part of the description. For example, individuals who have experienced loss respond differently and attach different meaning to the loss. This is critical for people in the human sciences to understand, in that there *is not a good way* to experience loss. Well, enough for the nod. It is important because it indicates agreement or recognition.

Rigor in Phenomenological Research.   Since some of us have difficulty remembering the concepts to evaluate qualitative research with,

I have tried—in addition to suggesting the phenomenological nod—to devise concepts that start with the letter "R" to indicate the criteria for Rigor. Perhaps you can think of additional ones to help you "R"emember.

- *Resonancy.* This concept or criterion indicates that the written interpretation of the meaning of the experience resonates with individuals. It sounds correct, fits in with past participation with the experience, explains a puzzle. It prompts familiar feelings and thoughts. Again, this may not apply to the entire text but a portion of it "rings true." It resonates.

- *Reasonableness.* Does the interpretation seem reasonable? Is it a possible explanation of the meaning of an experience? Also, were the means of attaining the material reasonable? Here we are asking for judicious reasoning. We are questioning the reasoning process. The researcher should have a carefully reasoned out rationale for the activities of the study, and people evaluating the study should be able to obtain a reasonable response to the question "Why?" for any part of the study.

- *Representativeness.* Does the study adequately represent the various dimensions of the lived experience? Was enough material concerning the phenomenon considered? This is where I think we need to understand the many avenues available to us in our quest for understanding. Figure 2.1 gives us some ideas where to listen and where to read so that the representation provides a broad variety of perspectives. "To the things themselves" does not translate to those ten interviews we have already discussed. The interviews are one of the "things." But if every time we would like to discuss the phenomenon with someone, we have ten steps to complete before doing so, we will lose the serendipitous conversation or the spontaneity of reading an article about our phenomenon on the front page of a newspaper. All is material, all are things. We must be careful that our requirement to go to the things themselves does not block our reaching them.

- *Recognizability.* Like resonancy, it rings a chord; yet within this criterion, individuals read the study who have not necessarily had the experience and they recognize certain aspects about an experience that they now become more acutely aware of, which leads to the next criterion.

- *Raised Consciousness.* This is a response to your study that engenders a focus toward and a gaining of understanding of an experience that the reader has not considered. Now brought to consciousness, the experience is seen fresh. One of my most recent examples of this was in a reading of "The Dwarf's Song" by Rainer Maria Rilke (1957).

  After hearing the poem, one of the members in the class said with surprise, "I never knew dwarfs had feelings." What is it like to be a dwarf? What meaning does this experience engender? The understanding is deeply enriched by including this poem as part of phenomenological material. This raised consciousness is both a criterion and simultaneously a very important aim of the phenomenological project. To become more human is to become more conscious of what we said previously of the "ordinary," "everydayness," and "the-taken-for-granted." We question our cherished beliefs. Going further, if everything *is* congruent with what you believed about the experience before you started, you might want to re-evaluate the reasonableness of your choices. When choosing phenomenological material, be careful that your choices do not become unconscious efforts to find a self-fulfilling prophecy. Some researchers embark on studies designed to demonstrate the "truth" of their own perceptions and interpretations. Not only researchers from the phenomenological perspective, but all researchers, must be vigilant of this tendency.

- *Readability.* A former student shared with me a letter of rejection from an editor for her phenomenological study saying that it was not abstract enough and I was reminded of Bohm's observation: "Everything is alive: what we call dead is an abstraction" (1980). Your study should read like an interesting conversation, and since we are attempting to understand experience, the writing should be understandable. Metaphors and analogies are useful aids to understanding. "Raising" something to an abstract level, it seems to me, is contrary to becoming more fully human. My personal view is that abstraction has somehow become equated with intellectualism. But what is your experience, for example, if you read an abstract poem where you have not a clue as to what the poet is saying? Indeed, readers often need to seek out a concrete interpretation of an interpretation of something that was concrete and has been made abstract! As I have mentioned before, I truly believe our studies not only belong in professional journals but in the popular literature people read (magazines, books, or other media). In these instances, the writing must be concrete, readable, and interesting.

- *Relevance.* Add relevance to the preceding sentence. Why do a study, even if your goal seems primarily to finish a degree, if it does not have relevance? Our studies should bring us close to our humanness, increase our consciousness, enable understanding, give us possible interpretations, offer us possible meaning, and guide us in our lives, personally and professionally. They should do nothing less for those we serve. Sometimes I mention "passion" as a variable in the selection of a study. When cruising through the multitude of unanswered questions, or experiences we do not understand, our mind should float until it is sparked. And that spark could ignite passion within us. There is no need to suffer through research. Seeking something to investigate that genuinely interests and excites you can make all the difference in your research experience. Consider relevance in a dual way: first, that the phenomenon is relevant to you, so that you can become absorbed beyond just your cognitive ability to do research, and second, that it is relevant to the field of human science and the human beings that such science serves.

- *Revelations.* In establishing criteria, it becomes obvious that they are not mutually exclusive categories. By now, if you have raised consciousness with a study that is relevant to the field, you undoubtedly have revealed something. This criterion, though, reminds us that often something was concealed and that we were able to find a deeper level of understanding. This reflects the philosophical idea that, behind or underneath what is revealed to us, we have considered what is being concealed or what wishes to be concealed.

- *Responsibility.* As researchers, we always have specific responsibilities. In the case of the phenomenological approach, we must always be aware of the ethical considerations of our study (see Chapter 9). Process consent, sensitivity to issues of conversations, and the reverence for authentic representation (as previously discussed in that chapter) are operative areas of our responsibility. Being true and being faithful to our participants and to the other phenomenological material we weave into our study are critical ethical concerns because we are so very close to human beings in the meaning and interpretation of our research.

Are there more R's? Perhaps a few—and then, add your own. The more perspectives you evaluate your study from, the more valuable and rigorous the process will be:

- *Richness.* A "rich" study is a full, embodied, multifaceted, multilayered, thoughtful, sensitive, impassioned description of a human experience; it will stir people. On the other hand, a "method" study is often an academic exercise. I'm sure you would prefer the first even if it seems more difficult. In the end, this richness will enrich you. Remember, one of the aims of phenomenology is to become more fully human.
- *Responsiveness.* How individuals, whether study participants or colleagues, respond to your study is important. Closely aligned with resonancy or recognizability, responsiveness can depart in a way here that is a *result* of your study. Are individuals moved to do something: to think through preconceptions or to follow through on your study? Are their imaginations stirred by different responses based on your descriptions and interpretations? Most important, Should they act on your research? If you can demonstrate that you have successfully met these criteria for rigor, then people should feel confident in trusting your work and using it toward the understanding of our humanness.

RESEARCH AND SOCIAL RESPONSIBILITY

Before closing here, I would like to mention again the need for our research to be socially responsive and meaningful. We should, as practitioners of human sciences, have this larger aim as our center.

The aim to respond to human needs, and the very civilization of humanity trumps anybody's idea of "approaches." Creatively seeking solutions goes beyond the status quo, and the discovery of new methods should be encouraged.

"That's not the way it's done" would seem to be an oxymoron for research. But it has implications. Art Buchwald, in an old column, satirized the research grant business. To paraphrase, he maintained that unless you can prove your research to be true, you can't get funded.

"It's never been done this way before, but if you can meet the criteria for rigor, why don't you try it" is not saying "anything goes," but it is providing opportunity. Not only should we be questing for new knowledge but *we should be questing for new ways of discovering knowledge and understanding.*

12

The Times Are Always Changing
Anecdotes, Journals, and Writing

This chapter continues to demonstrate the intertwining of the existential investigation and the importance of reflective writing. Journal entries and anecdotes are discussed as important means to understanding self and the other in the phenomenological process of being. In this chapter, we hear also from Chuck and Ray.

*J*ust as temporality, spatiality, corporeality, and relationality project us into what we call forward or the future, it is by the time we reflect upon it in the past.

So the present, past, and future can be all at once. Part of a story contains all these elements. My first anecdote, which could also be a journal entry, about Chuck, Ray, and myself now is in the past. Their travels, with mutual fears of abandonment emerging, is now in the present-day form and in the past as well.

They have moved to New Hampshire, where Chuck is the chairperson of a nursing department. This is probably a good career move.

Ray's future there is still uncertain. I am now Associate Dean of the Graduate Program in the school where Chuck was on faculty. So our paths have crisscrossed again.

At the moment, I am on a plane flying north to visit them. This will be a new way for us "to be" together.

How do I hold on to them, because they are so special to me? This trip is one way of doing that. We have spoken about everyday maintaining what we call "parallel analysis," and we are committed to writing a "role theory" book as co-authors. So is everything OK? Not at all. I miss them terribly, especially Chuck. I walk in the halls of my new school and his picture is on the wall and I feel a pang and so it goes.

Our relationship is being transformed. The situated context has changed. What is the meaning of this experience for me, and for Chuck and Ray? I will ask them and tell you about it shortly. The meaning is extremely complex. There is the apparent loss, and an onlooker might say, "So what? This happens every day; it is grist for the mill." *Exactly*. Because it happens every day, it is of interest to a phenomenologically oriented person—me.

It is the exact dynamic I described in Chapter 1. It is the experience of loss: the losses of years ago, the losses of last year, the losses that I have seen friends bear. So in seemingly ordinary lives, often some of the profoundest emotions, recalled and lived through once again in a different configuration, are felt almost "out of proportion." The meaning of the experience is, however, first what it appears to be and then what is concealed. "Out of proportion" would be the part that is concealed, and that being the case, it is often worthy of our attention.

Phenomenology as being in the world is a philosophy that seeks understanding of the meaning of being human. In this quest, we cannot *assume* that the response to a specific event is or is not appropriate. Responses lie in the recesses of each person's experience. That is why we are never finished. That is why one interview with an individual is hardly a sufficient attempt to understand a phenomenon.

My strongest criticism of some present-day phenomenological studies is that they are not "deep" enough or descriptive enough. Although we must probe judiciously, we can, for instance, ask people more often, "Could you give us an example" of whatever we are seeking to understand. Another question that seeks deeper understanding is, "Does this experience remind you of a similar experience?"

When doing hermeneutics or interpreting data, the more you think about the material, the greater your chances are of completing a hermeneutic circle, by going from part to whole or whole to part and then back again.

Doing this book concurrently with this story in my life has provided that opportunity for me. I have tried to be faithful to the story; at the same time, I know that what I've chosen to conceal is based on rational choice because of my specific audience.

This much, however, I can reveal because it is an excellent example of concealed meaning. Chuck and Ray's moving was a reliving of my own two sons growing up and appropriately separating from their mother. Like many mothers, not all, I found this separation painful, and anything that resembles it in a different context may very well stir up the feelings and the meanings from that other situation or the contingencies of my being.

Interpreting experience is a never-ending process. A thought came into my consciousness of the irony that children of 18 months of age or so are characteristically described as having "separation anxiety." Could it go back that far? If this type of thoughtfulness goes on in a study, its never-ending quality will become apparent.

It is the actual intentionality that makes thoughtful interpretation possible. Had I not embarked on this book would I have ever thought that Chuck and Ray's leaving was a reliving of a pre-oedipal separation anxiety for me, and for them as well?

This might not seem very dramatic, yet it is in this everyday world that we learn not to dismiss another person's feeling in a cursory way. A person's being and the meaning of that being is often responded to with phrases such as:

- You're making a mountain out of a molehill (cannot happen).
- You're overreacting (cannot happen).
- Don't make such a big deal of it (cannot help it).
- It's nothing, you'll feel better in a few days (cannot happen).

That is why we study meaning: to truly understand what an event or experience means to a person—not to us—but to the specific individual. And we need to reside with material given us, so that insights can occur that make our studies "meaningful" and provide us with description enabling us to understand what it means to be human. Only then can we respond to one another in an authentic way. Only then can we see the significance of an event to a person that is theirs, and not springing from our own anticipated response to an event.

The anecdotes about Chuck, Ray, and myself in this book are examples of an element of existential investigations. This kind of anecdotal material can appropriately be kept in a journal. If we do not write, we often tend to forget. In that "forgetting," we may often lose significant essences of an experience. Surely I would have "forgotten" that first ride to the airport.

So we must write in journals, we must record anecdotal material. The existential investigation comprising so much of the-life world must include ourselves as well. Self is part of every study. I've attempted to demonstrate this truism in this work, which is a study of phenomenology.

I am a part of this book. It would be impossible not to be. You are a part of this book. That too would be impossible not to be. Our experiences intertwine us in relationality. We need to capture them, though, or they will fly off like butterflies or perhaps, more painfully, crawl away like caterpillars.

We secure experiences in journals, films, photographs, conversations, notations in books such as novels and biographies, and in our writings about the experience in moments of reflection. If by chance, you would like to know more about this Chuck and Ray thread, that is all to the good because it is here to demonstrate the significance of the ordinary.

The visit was a roller coaster. The house that they just had bought was put back on the market because Ray had not found employment. On Saturday, he planned to return to Miami and his former job as a teacher. Sunday, this all *appeared* settled. Monday, the house was off the market, Ray was staying, and that *appeared* settled. It is now three weeks later, and the house is back on the market.

I have asked each of them to write an anecdote of this experience, so that we might better understand their perspectives.

The Meaning of Moving
Charles J. Beauchamp

What is this move all about? A question I have asked myself, liter-ally a million times. And as I write this piece, I am still unsure. I am beginning to feel comfortable with the ambiguity of this life-event, and the reality that I may never know. At different times and in dif-ferent ways I experience the entire situation very differently. The meaning of the move doesn't change, but the experience of it does. The things that excited me about the move at times are the very things that I dread; and paradoxically the things that I dreaded are the very things that excite me. When I was there, I wished to be here. Now that I am here, I frequently wish to be there. Will I ever be happy here, instead of there?

The answers to these questions don't seem as important to me as the questions themselves. I have begun to realize that toward the end of my days there, in Miami, it seemed as though I stopped ask-ing questions. And since I've moved here, to New Hampshire, I have done nothing but ask questions. How could I have done this to Tri-cia? How could I have done this to Ray? How could I have done this to my students, patients, and colleagues? Why am I doing this to myself? As I reflect upon this move, I have come to the realization that the meaning is reflected in the questions or the questioning, not in any of the answers.

What then are these questions or questioning about? I have found meaning in this move by asking questions, not by answering them. In Miami, I had begun to have more answers than questions. I now realize that questions and questioning serve as a propelling force within my life. Upon further examination of this move, I have also found that Tricia, Ray, students, patients, colleagues, as well as myself, were the very source of the questions which spurred this move on.

Did they then do this to me? Or, did I do this to them? Am I living It's a Wonderful Life *or* Nightmare on Elm Street? *Did I need to move? Could I have stayed? Could I go back? What is this move all about?*

When Fiction Becomes Reality: The Move
Raymond Klimasewski, Jr.

I thought I was ready for a change; I really needed a change. It didn't have to be New Hampshire, but New Hampshire was fine. Chuck really needed to move, and wanted to move. I wanted to be supportive and thought the move would be beneficial for myself as well. Everything about leaving Miami for New Hampshire seemed to be perfect, except the weather. I was willing to give up the year-round sunshine for new opportunities.

Opportunity, as I reflect, appeared to be at the center of this move. A great opportunity for Chuck, one that would also provide opportunities for me. I had always thought of opportunity as an emerging situation that presents with hope and happiness for what lies ahead. This move started out with great hope and happiness, but soon turned into a trying time full of turmoil. As in my life situations, nothing turned out as planned.

I planned on having a peaceful summer, full of fun on Cape Cod; instead we spent the summer miserably trying to orchestrate a move. What began as an adventure ripe with opportunity, soon turned into an agitating situation with limited options. Many clichés come to mind when I reflect back, like: "If it seems to be too good to be true, it is"; "Always get everything in writing"; "It's service after the sale that counts"; "You can never really go back"; and "When troubled times occur, you'll find out who your true friends are."

Am I happy? I don't know! I'm happier than I was a month ago. But I am probably not as happy as I was a year ago. The opportunities are not as they were described to us. But, other opportunities that we, or I, never thought of have emerged. It has been these unexpected opportunities that have provided hope for the future and moments of happiness during this time. The authors of the factious opportunities are fading into their rightful places in their own created worlds. While my life is brighter with the wonderful people I have me along with the comfort and of my "true friends." Thank you Tricia, my true friend!

Again perceptual differences emerge. The reader can dwell with all the alternative *ways of perceiving* an "objective" event. You might feel the tugging at heartstrings as well.

13

Paler Shades of Black and White

Questions and Tentative Answers

This chapter presents additional material in our quest to understand phenomenology. These questions and answers come from seminar and class groups and thus are grounded in the life-world.

There are, however, no definitive answers; there is more to every answer, and then there is probably more to the question.

I would like to share with you some questions and answers from recent seminars that I gave. Although I say "gave," the seminar was a joint undertaking of a group of people who were interested in the phenomenological perspective in the human sciences. My answers are not necessarily the "right" answers. I perceived each question and gave a subjective response. These interchanges are brief but demonstrate another way of probing.

During the first day of the seminar, I acknowledged that often questions that individuals have when attending a seminar do not get addressed, so each day I asked for homework. The participants were

to write down any question, and I would attempt to answer it the following day. (I've read that sometimes women feel odd dining alone
in a restaurant. Well, if that should happen to you, just bring 20 index
cards—with questions on them—to dinner and enjoy thoughtfully
conversing with them.) The following morning, we would go over
the questions, because in many instances, the content was very much
related. Other participants also contributed insights to the questions.

Perhaps you will find some of your own questions here. Perhaps
you might answer them differently. Please let me know.

QUESTIONS FROM STUDENTS

Carol Germain: How do we write creatively while at the same
time trying to be acceptable to the realities of the publishing
world of nursing science?

A: Journals tend to be very strict in a quest for formalistic style.
As a peer reviewer, as I imagine many of you are for many journals, you know the concrete, tight criteria that you are asked to
judge a manuscript on. It seems now that the longer your list of
references is, the more merit your article has.

I would suggest contributing chapters in free-thinking edited
books and seeking publishers who want something creative or,
as they may put it, "hot." You need to write to what is topical
and meaningful today or, as Popper has suggested, refute
through research what is "taken for granted." Carol, you're writing in the "women's experience" book and that will give you a
full chapter; and don't forget "Green Leaves, Sour Grapes, and
Writing for *Mirabella*" (Preface in this book).

Martha From: How do I know when I have captured the essence
of the experience? How deep is deep enough?

A: This is the time for the phenomenological nod. Bring back your
description to the participants and ask them, "Have I expressed
the experience the way it is for you?" Collaborative consultation
is also good—ask others, "Does this resonate with your experience or not?" "Deep"—I suppose a person can always probe
more—but time is a consideration. Deep is when the study has

captured something. It becomes relevant. Deep does not necessarily mean finished. There are different levels of depth. But I will once again reiterate, deep is not when you have described a situated context of life-worlds embedded in contingency in a sentence. Deep has some pragmatic considerations with a value of meaningfulness in our everyday being-in-the-world.

Karen Moore Schaefer: How does reflective thinking relate to phenomenology?

A: The activity is part of hermeneutic phenomenological study, the attempt to grasp the essential meaning of something. The thinking is more direct—intended toward something, resides with it as an experience. Van Manen (1990) suggests using the life-world existential to guide our reflecting. Lived experience can only be grasped by reflectively thinking in the past. In the moment, reflecting on it changes the experience.

Catherine Nass Kotecke: If language is the key to phenomenology, how can we approach people who do not have language (i.e., deaf/dumb people)? People who have different language meanings?

A: Language as just verbal speaking, I believe, is a metaphor for communication. Of course, people who are deaf may need to be interviewed with a person familiar with sign language, who can immediately translate to you. Same with Braille for blind people. I think that we often tend to become discouraged when we cannot communicate verbally with someone in our own language, not only those who may be deaf or blind but also those from different socioeconomic levels or cultures. This is a good question because it reminds us of the "forgotten" people. Remember when we said that a criterion in our studies is the willingness to talk about the experience. That needs to be interpreted as the willingness to communicate in any way an individual is able to.

Sara Lauterbach: Having used Heidegger in my dissertation, and being aware of the current critique of Heidegger, I am still thinking about this issue. It is bothersome to me that Heidegger's political and intellectual life are so discrepant. What do you think about this?

A: Jung says we all have a shadow. If we are good people in a general sense, our shadow carries our dark traits but we go on as being good. Not knowing for sure, there are so many issues here, I have thought that the work Heidegger did prior to these accusations was the good Heidegger. If later, his dark shadow took over (as in psychopathology or cowardice or whatever) it doesn't seem to negate his work prior to that.

As a generality, many geniuses were schizophrenics or had psychotic breaks. We have mentioned oftentimes the essential values of the situated context in the quest to understand the meaning of experience. Richard Rorty (1992) calls this the *role of contingency*. So like the situated context, the role of contingency will influence tremendously our perceptions and our actions. In Rorty (1992), contingency means the accident and chance of where we find ourselves "being." Contingency then influences our commitments, virtues, and mistakes.

Philosophers as well as researchers have given much thought and attention to the works of Heidegger. This is no small matter because Heidegger's works on being have made him one of the most influential philolsophers of the century. Yet, it has become known that the philosopher of "being and becoming through caring" has been implicated in the Nazi regime. Rorty interprets this phase of Heidegger's life as a way of illustrating the role of contingency. Knowing that most of the philosopher's writings were written before Hitler's rise to power, Rorty cites the fates of accident and chance in forming our commitments, virtues, and mistakes and amplifies that Heidegger was in a situated context. He poses the possibility that instead of staying in Germany and giving nebulous speeches on the new German Reality, he could have, as a matter of chance, fallen in love with a Jewish student, left his wife and country, and taken exile elsewhere. His ideas would have been more or less the same, but his professional life would have been more consistent with his philosophical beliefs. Instead, as Rorty (1992) states, he wound up "a coward, a liar, and the greatest philosopher of the century" (p. 57).

Zane Wolf: How does the phenomenological movement in nursing fit in the larger world context of phenomenology?

A: If nurse researchers have embarked on inquiry as to the meaning of experience, being-in-the-world, and what it means to be human, we have a tremendous potential to add knowledge to the larger context of the world of understanding. As you know, we are with people everywhere, every day, and according to the American Nurses' Association, we exist to diagnose and treat human responses to almost everything. So if we learn to understand these responses, then I think it would be a tremendous contribution. Also because of where we are situated, nurses are present from before birth to after death with people in all their vulnerabilities, vicissitudes, and strengths. I believe we're an ideal profession to contribute to the larger context of understanding being. Perhaps more so than any other profession.

Mary Ann Dailey: What is the best way to explain a qualitative proposal to a quantitative mind?

A: Explaining to a person with an open mind is easy, and there is plenty written about the differences between logical positiveness and phenomenology. To a closed mind, perhaps ask if the person would read what's new in mathematical probability theory and also see or read *Fried Green Tomatoes*. And that is the difference.

Marilyn Meder: My major question deals with justifying the worthiness of my study. I am interested in the experiences of African-American nursing students.

A: You're asking about the worthiness of studying a subculture of nursing at present, culturally and socially. Well, what is it like for them? Do we care? Should we care? I think there is a preunderstanding or preconception that their experience might be different from other nursing students, again depending on their situated context. If there is a "possibility of being" that includes being discriminated against, for instance, then what do you think? This is why we exist, to become closer to human experience.

Susan Davis:
1. How do you select the sample and know when the number you've selected is adequate?

2. How do you develop your interview questions?

3. I've read Guba and Lincoln's book and the section on reliability and validity but am unsure how to ensure these qualities in my study.

A: 1. I had answers here but they were the regular answers. These questions are now answered somewhat differently within this work, many times because of our dialogic conversations. However, these "kinds" of questions now I would hope you would answer from the perspective of the experience and the direction that your participants, your attentiveness, and your raised consciousness propel you toward.

2. Interview questions—You are going to have a dialogic conversation. Ask one or two questions: "What is it like to become a mother?" The rest is to further clarify and obtain examples, "Could you tell me more, I'm not sure I understand"—remember you are trying to grasp the meaning of an experience as described by another.

3. The qualities that Guba and Lincoln use for reliability and validity for the academic setting are fine to use. (I like the ones suggested in this book better!) Phenomenology should be judged in my opinion by resonancy—does it ring with truth, familiarity, and possibility (see Chapter 11 of this volume).

Jane Brennan: How does one select among the various phenomenological approaches—descriptive, interpretive, etc.?

A: It depends on your purpose. However, there are some people including myself that think all experience is interpreted even if it is called descriptive. We are always engaged in interpreting realities. We never see anything in a pure way because we have an active unconscious. However, knowing that our descriptions have a selective interpretation to them assists us in using care. What I think is critical is to stay as faithful to what was interpreted to you, others' interpreted experience, the subjectivity of the teller, so to speak, before you attempt to interpret the experience.

A STUDENT ANSWERS QUESTIONS

Students can often answer questions very well. The following phenomenological material, in the form of questions and answers, was written by Susan Manter, who had been unable to attend a class session. She later listened to a tape of the class and then reviewed her notes as follows:

Q: Summarize briefly the preceding week.

A: According to Rilke, being is going inside with intensity. Phenomenology looks for the subjective differences of individuals. The end point of such research should be writing . . . a narrative. To understand the phenomenon, you must start with personal experience. Sometimes the reason for choosing that particular phenomenon is an intense personal interest. Therefore, it helps to understand yourself and your own experience. This is why a personal journal is critical . . . to remember the thoughts that flit through your mind. If they aren't written down, then they are often lost and not regained. The phenomenological process raises consciousness. But it is a concrete action, not an abstract theory. It involves doing. Certain assumptions predispose the phenomenon. These are "taken-for-granted" beliefs. They are not tested or proven, but are so much a part of our everyday lives that they are taken for truths. We all base our behaviors on these assumptions. Therefore, looking at our assumptions is very important before beginning research. Bracketing, or the setting aside of recognized ideas and beliefs from our personal lives, is imperative and should go on constantly. This way, we won't read anything into others' lived experiences that comes from our own. This is a difficult thing to do and we must constantly remind ourselves of it.

A research method is only a way of studying certain kinds of questions. But the method is not the important thing in phenomenology. The question itself is the starting point, and many ways of finding the answers can be used. It does involve the personal experiences of human beings. It comes from the perspective of human science, which includes thoughts, feelings, actions, beliefs, values, and consciousness from the human world. Human science studies persons that have consciousness that act purposefully in and on the world by creating objects of meaning as the expression of how we live in the world. Once you arrive at a question of interest, it will always be with you. Data are found in surprising nooks and crannies, and we must always be on the lookout. The question comes from lived experience, and lived experience goes on constantly. The question will guide the way you go about collecting data (the method). You become the question and are constantly conscious of it. This is not the sort of research you do on Saturday morning. You must be always on, always alert. It is not whimsical research. There are always voices speaking to you and material that is relevant to all around you. Anytime, you can pick up on something that increases understanding. The open approach is the only way to truly obtain the experiences of others.

You must be always open to new information. When the research is finished, and there should be an ending date or time, the results will inform others.

Q: What is pedagogy?

A: According to van Manen, pedagogy is the activity of teaching, parenting, educating, or generally living with children, that requires constant practical acting in concrete situations and relations. Actually it refers to the teaching, or educating, of children.

Q: What is the connection between researching and writing?

A: By writing the results of research, the unconscious becomes conscious and it gives experience a form of expression. Writing allows you to enter a stream-of-consciousness experience, whether it is your own or someone else's. It allows the results to be read and experienced again and again, which brings depth of understanding.

Q: What is method idolatry?

A: Method idolatry occurs when the method becomes more important than the research itself. Methodologists are those who have an ideology of methods, and this causes them to focus on the technique. In phenomenology, it is important to not be confined by methods. This tends to formalize or categorize experience, and the intense meaning is lost along the way.

Q: What does it mean to be rational?

A: Van Manen states that human science is rationalistic, in that it operates on the assumption that human life can be made intelligible and accessible to our reason. If we are rational, we can understand the world by remaining in thoughtful and conversational relationship to it. Things will not be crystal clear, but the concept that living is a shared experience makes our lives understandable and intelligible, especially through our language. We take the world as we find it, try to make reflected experience explicit, and attempt to seek meaning. These are rational actions.

14

With A Lot of Help from My Friends
The Book Pauses

This chapter brings this book to a pause. If the book stimulates discussion and raises questions, the work continues.

If you understand the meaning of the phenomenological perspective in a "user friendly" way, I've accomplished some "thing" that gives meaning to me. I hope this text as an examplar gives meaning to your endeavors in the murky world, as you, too, attempt to find the meaning of being—a task of no small consequence.

I wish for you many ways to find the meaning of being in our everyday worlds.

When people discuss phenomenology as a research approach, they often ask me, "How do I know when I'm finished?" Once an individual's intentionality is directed toward a particular experience, the phenomenon seems to appear in a way that could characteristically be conceptualized as "always there," and a researcher becomes aware of the "always more." So how does a person stop the process of gathering material for a study?

This question is also applicable to this book. I have turned toward the phenomenon of the study of experience, and the manuscript could conceivably continue to grow. I could keep responding to appearances. Since the publisher expects the finished manuscript this week, I asked my editor, Allan Graubard, the same question about completion that students ask me when they are doing research from this perspective. I wrote this inquiry in letter form, between other items of business, because the knowing of the incompleteness of this book is coinciding with the deadline. He answered on my "machine" and as so often, very wisely: "When a book is printed, it definitely is never finished, it lives, it continues, and even lives after us."

I feel understood (coincidentally the aim of phenomenology), and I am more at ease with the "unfinished" version. So how to stop? Later in the day, I spoke to Allan on the phone because, like students, I still needed a concrete answer. He asked me how many pages I had written and I answered, and he replied that was more than sufficient. So that is how you end that phase and go on to do something else with the material.

Though a person might question, as a standard, something that seems arbitrary—length of manuscript, a due date, whatever of life's contingencies—it still remains a good answer.

I often suggest to students when they ask that same question, to consider when they want to complete this *phase* of the study, implying that the study is not finished. Unlike a researcher who tests a hypothesis, obtains an answer, and in some way, has closure at least for that particular question, research grounded by phenomenology is never "finished."

"Being" in the world continues and is "always more." That truth certainly applies to this work, and I suggest that you use this understanding when asking the question about your own research.

Any study of lived experience is ongoing, ever changing, and responsive to the vicissitudes of the situated context. However, you need to pause at some place and begin to write and then stop writing, guided by a due date, or number of pages. This does not imply completion, for once "attuned," you will most likely continue your work in one way or another. The researcher and the writer are not separate entities. The gaze and intentionality of this project are written in my being-in-the-world. If and when I finally send the manuscript to be published, I will still be writing it. I know this because I started this book metaphorically in 1982 (Munhall, 1982). My being has led to this book as part of a process and will not end with the mailing of a manuscript.

I am impassioned by ideas I read, and reflect on them as regards phenomenology. The appearances in my life are evidence of this, the writings, the research, the Saturday seminars, the summer workshops, and the requests to conduct a course in this approach. I am anything but finished. In the moment, I grow in consciousness.

For my students, I attempt to demonstrate the continuity of their beliefs as integral to their being, integral to their humanness, and not something *out* there. Their research is not separate from them, how could it be? The phenomenon they choose to study alters their perceptual lens to capture the appearance. Sometimes it is purposeful; oftentimes, it occurs serendipitously and we are surprised to find "it" wherever. Study from a phenomenological perspective resides within a person, some have said, living with the person. For me, it has taken up residence within me. This is not to say it is always a peaceful residence, since I often seem to be justifying this way of being. I hope some of that justification becomes clear within this work. For now, I offer the justification that phenomenology as philosophy would argue vehemently against the following all-too-true assumptions of higher education:

> *From a doctoral examination "What is the task of all higher educa-*
> *tion?" To turn men into machines. "What are the means?" Man*
> *must learn to be bored. "How is that accomplished?" By means of*
> *the concept of duty. "Who serves as the model?" The philogist: he*
> *teaches grounding. "Who is the perfect man?" The civil servant.*
> *"Which philosophy offers the highest formula for the civil servant?"*
> *Kant's the civil servant as thing-in-itself raised up to be judge over*
> *the civil servant as phenomenon.*
>
> *Nietzsche*
> *(p. 125 in Siderberg)*

Phenomenology as philosophy and not as ideology is in sharp contrast to what might be the purpose of higher education. The purpose of higher education is not to create "model" citizens, since such a

condition would secure the world as it presently exists or is propelling forward to. The purpose rather "should be to assist individuals in being-more-fully-human and to emancipate and liberate
individuals from their preconceptions." The phenomenologist is
even able to see danger in shared meanings that might assume a
"reality" and appear to transcend our individual participation.

So how could a work on phenomenology be even conceivably con-
cluded when as a philosophical work, it questions its own presuppositions? The phenomenologist reflects not only on the meaning of a
particular human experience, but on the meaning of meaning within
a situated context. Shared bonds of meaning are essential for our being human, yet must be evaluated for the underlying meaning of
sharing. The question of meaning always reflects back on the meaning of that sharing, and so may seem paradoxical. Yet it is critical that
meaning not become confused with ideology.

Each of us should hold precious, our own individual interpretation of reality. We need not abandon that, in the face of others
sharing a different interpretation. Questions then are to the self,
and self-reflection may yield the real-life everyday experience of
discontinuity. We are not all alike. We do not perceive experience
in the same way, and it is certainly not the goal of phenomenological research to produce one shared meaning of an experience that
represents *all* humans.

How impossible that would be. What the phenomenologist can
produce for us is an interpretation of a human experience in a particular situated context that *may* help us understand what it means to
be human under those particular conditions in those contingencies
for some individuals.

The phenomenological nod gives credence to the familiar aspects
of the description, but often we may not be familiar with the description. Unfamiliarity is good. It means perhaps a new window from
which to perceive a phenomenon. So both are a part of the experience in phenomenology—shared meaning and unfamiliar meaning.

When we read an interpretation of an experience that we are unable to relate to or understand, yet it was "that way" for others, we
should not dismiss it. This is often where we must reflect on our own
biases, assumptions, and ideologies. I have often heard interpretations of experiences dismissed because the interpretation did not

match the reader's own reality. Of course, most of you recognize this "resistance" to a new interpretation as the greatest obstacle to change, or in this case, reperceiving an experience, in a different way that places a crack in your foundational beliefs or assumptions about being in the world.

That is why I have tried to weave a human experience throughout this work. In Chapter 4, on unknowing, there is a discussion of intersubjectivity. As you have read this book, our subjectivities have become intertwined and reading in itself occurs in an intersubjective world. So what is said about unknowing is applicable to this work as well. The idea of "knowing" something with complete certainty, I propose, leads to premature closure.

There is always more to know, there is always an alternative and in this particular moment, now past, there is no end. The temporality of being is ever changing, and we need even more to be attentive and wide awake to our everyday world. In that ordinary day lie mysteries of being human whose meanings are lost to us unless we turn to them with wonder. I believe nothing is meaningless, literally. If the ordinary is translated as "nothing's new," then the ordinary will be meaningless.

Individuals apparently need meaning. It is why we choose to live. Phenomenology offers to us a way to come upon that meaning, and if we are open to those ways, never finished, we are always being and becoming. We are always coming upon meaning, the meaning being human.

Before leaving, I would like to re-emphasize where you might find examples of phenomenological writing, including the next chapter by Lucy Warren and Sarah Lauterbach's study in Munhall and Oiler's (1993) *Nursing Research: A Qualitative Perspective. In Women's Experience* (in press) offers ten additional chapters. Also, I hope many of you will have seen this book as a phenomenology, an attempt to understand phenomenology itself.

I certainly would be amiss if I did not share with you that my experience with Chuck and Ray now includes many airport arrivals and departures, all fraught with meaning. However, meaning is always changing, so I am more awake and attentive to the character of nuance. My "travels now with Chuck" include much telephoning and yet a deep abiding concern and love that endures. This love is very meaningful to me. The love, this book, my attempts to understand, have all been inspired by many people, in and out of this book and as in the acknowledgments, I thank them. And, I thank you, the reader, and do hope you engaged in dialogue with the perceptions presented here. For that is all they are.

15

A Study as Exemplar

The Experience of Feeling Cared for: A Phenomenological Perspective

Lucy D. Warren

The aim of this work based on the phenomenological perspective was to de-termine what people mean when they say they "felt cared for." It was assumed that knowing this would help nurses understand an important aspect of the phenomenon of caring.

The phenomenological investigation included the collection of data from my personal experiences, from etymological sources, from experiential descrip-tions from healthy adults obtained during serial open-ended interviews, and

About the Author: Lucy D. Warren, RN, EdD is currently an Associate Professor at Kean College of New Jersey. She has taught nursing for many years, teaching pedi-atrics at Columbia University's School of Nursing for 10 years before getting post-graduate training in psychotherapy, and teaching at Pace University before coming to Kean. Lucy combines her interests in pediatrics and psychiatry and works as a mental health consultant to the nursing staff at Children's Specialized Hospital in Toms River, New Jersey. She is involved in the planning stages of a study that will use the phenomenological method to learn about home care of children. Lucy is also ac-tive in the American Cancer Society and Sigma Theta Tau. When not working, her interests include her family, their dogs, and the out-of-doors.

from descriptions and depictions found in literature, art, and music. Based on reflections on the data, a phenomenological writing about the experience of feeling cared for was composed.

Please search yourselves for resources to deal helpfully with others like us (a mother whose 17-year-old daughter died in an automobile accident). Seek ways to make the few moments available for deeply troubled persons times of healing rather than destruction. Plan ways of staffing your facilities with people who are full of heart and wise in the administration of compassion. We need caring so desperately. (cited in Reilly, 1978, p. v)

Caring has been identified as the core of nursing (Watson, 1979), and the essence and central focus for nursing decisions, practices and goals (Leininger, 1981). Benner (1984, p. 170) has stated that the phenomenon of care plays the central role in all examples of excellent nursing care. Such claims made by respected nurse researchers are supported by their qualitative studies, but there are still many unanswered questions about the concepts of care and caring. The simple fact that there are so many words and phrases associated with the concepts makes the challenge of understanding them a formidable one.

This phenomenological study focused on the experience of "feeling cared for." The method of phenomenology was chosen because while doing a pilot study and interviewing several people, I found that data emerged not only from the interviews but from books they or I had read, from art they had seen, from music, theater, and even from colleagues, friends, and relatives who had heard what I was studying. Phenomenology was a method that would allow for the collection of data wherever it could be found, whether subjective or objective, without predetermined biases as to how to focus the study. So, while I did interview ten healthy adults in depth and over time, in order to arrive at a phenomenological writing about feeling cared for, I also used as data my own life experiences and personal journal reflections, anecdotal descriptions from anyone who offered them, etymological sources, literary and artistic sources, all in order to more fully understand the phenomenon (see Figure 15.1).

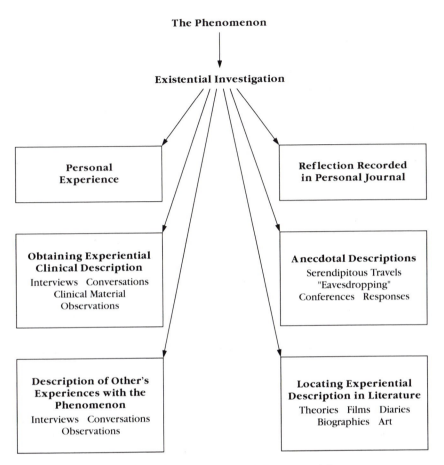

Figure 15.1.   The Phenomenon and Existential Investigation.

The actual data collected in phenomenological research can be so rich and full of meaning that I have included numerous verbatim examples of the data. Initially, specific themes were identified only in the participants' interviews, primarily so I would know when conducting additional interviews with new participants would be unlikely to add new data. The other sources of data (personal experiences, etymological sources, and literary and artistic sources) are presented without theme identification. The personal experiences and the examples from literature and art were recorded or collected throughout the period of the study with the only requirement being that they depicted cared-for-ness for the person suggesting them. The etymological sources were considered complete when the appropriate words or phrases had been located and defined.

After the data are presented, the identified themes are presented. Finally, the result of phenomenological reflection and phenomenological writing based on the data collection is presented. This writing, albeit very simple in its final form, is the culmination of three years of my living in an attitude of thoughtful attention to and ofttimes specific study of the experience of feeling cared for.

ASSUMPTIONS AND BIASES RELATED TO THE STUDY OF THE PHENOMENON

My interest in the topic of caring stemmed from a belief that human beings need both to *be* cared for and to *feel* cared for in order to thrive. The famous separation studies done in English orphanages after World War II (Ainsworth, 1966) and the Harlow monkey studies (1959) showed that living beings must not only receive adequate physical care in order to grow and thrive, but must also receive what could be termed emotional or psychological care . . . they must *feel* cared for. Ainsworth (1966) reported on numerous studies done on London children separated from their mothers during and after World War II, which found that although basic physical needs were met, the children suffered serious long-term consequences from the effects of separation from their mothers. The children studied were found to be deficient in their abilities to use language and abstraction and to develop and maintain meaningful interpersonal relationships (1966, p. 341).

During this same time period, H. F. Harlow, an animal psychologist, was studying the effects of withdrawing all social, tender, loving contacts from infant monkeys (1959). Harlow discovered that while the infant monkeys survived with wire or cloth surrogate mothers, food, and water, they were unable as adults to interact socially or sexually with other monkeys. Based on these kinds of studies, the effects of absence of nurturing and feeling cared for are assumed to cause serious psychological problems. A major assumption of this study was that feeling cared for has powerful and positive outcomes for people, increasing feelings of self-worth and self-esteem.

I also believe that nurses need to be concerned with care and caring as a vital component of nursing, and there is a growing body of nursing literature that discusses different caring activities, attitudes, factors, and assumptions (Griffin, 1983; Leininger, 1981; Watson, 1979, 1985). Specifically, Jean Watson (1979, 1985) developed a list of ten carative factors based on seven carative assumptions, and Madeleine Leininger (1981) described caring practices related to health in various cultures. Because the nature of phenomenological research requires that the researcher begin the study with as few biases and theories as possible, I purposely refrained from doing an in-depth literature review before beginning the data collection. These works were reviewed in depth after the data collection was well under way.

EXISTENTIAL INVESTIGATION

Van Manen said that this stage of existential investigation requires that the researcher stand both in the fullness of life and in the midst of shared situations, remembering all the while to explore the category of lived experience in as many of its aspects as possible (1984, p. 40). The following pages describe the data collected during this stage of existential investigation of feeling cared for.

Recording of Personal Experiences

When I thought about personal experiences of feeling cared for, the first memory was one of being a child of four or five and having just had my tonsils taken out. I was in a hospital bed, having recently returned from the operation, and I woke up feeling very nauseated and proceeded to "throw up" on the pillow and sheets as I lay in bed. I was horrified at what I'd done, for I thought I'd made a real mess and was sure I would incur someone's wrath for having done so. As it turned out, some wonderful woman came into the room and when I started to apologize, she quickly reassured me that it was quite OK, that she'd change the sheets for me right away and that I would probably begin to feel better *because* I had thrown up. This experience had always seemed to me to represent the best of nursing in my own life experience and now it represented for me a clear and vivid personal experience of "feeling cared for."

Additional memories of feeling cared for centered around little things . . . one of my parents sitting on my bedside when I was sick as a child with some minor illness, my parents bringing a gift on their return from a trip, letters or calls from family and friends that seemed to come at just the right moment.

Recent experiences center around times of stress due to illness or the challenges of being a partner and parent . . . times when my husband would "be present" for me, often just to listen to my fears or concerns or irrational ravings if I was upset; times when he would accompany me to a difficult doctor's appointment, or hold me, or fight with me when I was needing to fight, or support me in my work when it meant less time or energy for him.

It was my experiences with my husband in fact that made me begin to question my understanding of this thing called caring. I had always thought I was a very caring person. I was, after all, a nurse . . . I like to keep a home and do all sorts of motherly, wifely things . . . but these things weren't always what he needed. They were things I wanted to give, but not things that ended making him feel cared for. He wanted my presence and what he called "relatedness" more than a clean house and clothes, and I couldn't always give that . . . so I began to realize that maybe I didn't understand this thing called caring so well and maybe there was a lot to learn about what made one person feel cared for as opposed to another person. It began to be clear to me that there was a distinct difference between "caring for" and feeling cared for.

Additional personal experiences could be shared but would not add as much to the richness of the data as would the examples from the participants. A journal of these personal experiences and reflections was kept and often referred to. I found that keeping such a journal was helpful especially in that it offered a concrete way of reminding me where my particular biases might be. As the phenomenological reflection and writing began, I found that journal entries stopped, as if the writing became my personal expression of all that I had collected (a synthesis of sorts).

Tracing Etymological Sources

In this study, I was interested in tracing the sources of the words "care" and "feeling" and also in the source of the phrase "feeling cared for." According to the *Oxford English Dictionary*, "caring" comes from the Old English and Gothic words *carian* and *kara.* The noun comes from *kara* and means "grief, lament, or sorrow." According to the *Dictionary of Word Origins* (Shipley, 1945), the original meanings of the word, "sorrow or lament," shifted to "trouble," then to "troubling yourself, taking trouble," hence to "taking care, being careful."

Griffin (1983) discusses the many uses and meanings of the words care and caring and their evolution. She described the earliest use of the noun a little differently. She said that the noun care meant charging the mind with concern or attention as in to "attend to this matter with due care." Later addition of the word "for" changed the sense of attending with care to one of "regard arising from desire or liking." The word then evolved to mean a sense of protection for, as seen in the statement "he is in the care of a nurse." Griffin (1983) stated that this sense of the word has become obsolete although care does still indicate a mind that is thoughtful toward or attentive to something or someone.

In the verbal form, care, from *carian,* refers to the idea "to trouble oneself." This usage indicates that the subject has concern for or feels interest in the object, provides, or looks after, has a liking or inclination toward the object. Griffin (1983, p. 315) concludes from the etymology of the word *care* that although there is no one meaning for the word, the "general family of meanings are all related to the notion of caring in one of three senses: attention to or concern for; responsibility for or providing for; regard, fondness, or attachment."

An ancient parable of care is seen occasionally in the literature about care and is recorded here, as myths or parables often capture better than dictionaries the real meaning of a word or concept. This version of the parable is as follows:

Once Care was crossing a river. She saw some clay on the ground beneath her feet. She thoughtfully and carefully took up a piece and began to shape it. While she was meditating on what she had made,

Jupiter came by. Care asked Jupiter to give it spirit and this he gladly did. But when Care wanted her name to be bestowed upon it, he forbade this and demanded that it be called Jupiter instead. While Care and Jupiter were arguing, Earth arose and desired her own name conferred on the creature, since she had furnished it with part of her body. They asked Saturn to be their arbiter, and he made the following just decision: "Since you, Jupiter, gave it its spirit, you shall receive that spirit as its death. Since you, Earth, are the source of its body, you shall receive its body at its death. And since you, Care, shaped it, you must take care of it and attend to it throughout its lifetime. But I, I will call it Homos or Human. (Dvorkin, Himmelstein, & Lesnick, cited in Constantino, 1988, p. 74)

This myth about Care would seem to support Griffin's claim that care refers to a general set of meanings: concern for, responsibility for, and attachment to.

Having discussed the source of the words care and caring, it is relevant also to trace the origins of the word "feeling," since it is a crucial part of the phenomenon under study. *Webster's Ninth Collegiate Dictionary* defines feeling as a noun that first appeared in the twelfth century, and it lists eight different meanings. The first meaning relates to touch, to the basic physical sensation that occurs when the skin with its sense organs comes into contact with something. The second meaning has to do with an emotional state or reaction to something. The third meaning is the undifferentiated background of one's awareness considered apart from any identifiable sensation, perception, or thought, the overall quality of one's awareness, or conscious recognition. The last four meanings in order are: capacity to respond emotionally; the character ascribed to something (atmosphere); the quality of a work of art that embodies and conveys the emotion of the artist; and finally, "a feel for . . . ."

For the purposes of this work, the first definition for feeling, the one having to do with touch, is not relevant unless one thinks of it in terms of its idiomatic use, of "being or feeling touched" by some experience. This way of using the word "touched" is really a way of saying one "felt a feeling," usually a positive one, although the feeling itself is not specified.

The other definitions for feeling all relate to some psychological or emotional experience. Some psychologists believe that one reason psychotherapy is so utilized and so relevant in our time is because it helps people to focus on feelings, and as such, does something that no other groups did until the popular support groups of recent years. Rollo May (1969), in *Love and Will*, said that relationships of love begin with a feeling of care or concern for another. He went on to discuss his views on feeling:

> *The new basis for care is shown by the interest of psychologists and philosophers in emphasizing* feeling *as the basis of human existence. We now need to establish feeling as a legitimate aspect of our way of relating to reality. When William James says, "Feeling is everything," he means not that there is nothing* more *than feeling, but that everything starts there. Feeling commits one, ties one to the object, and ensures action. But in the decades after James made this "existentialist" statement, feeling became demoted and was disparaged as merely subjective. Reason . . . was the guide to the way issues were to be settled. We said "I feel" as a synonym for "I vaguely believe," when we didn't know—little realizing that we cannot know except as we feel. (May, 1969, p. 303)*

Complementing Rollo May's thoughts on feelings is a work by James Hillman (1979), in which he traced the history of attitudes toward feelings up to recent times when it was left to the newly developing field of psychology to support the study of the importance of feelings to human life. According to Hillman, despite psychology's focus on feelings, it is still very difficult for most adults in our time to easily discuss "feelings." It's as if we do not have the language or the words to describe such states and we end up experiencing what T. S. Eliot (1943, p. 31) described as "the general mess of imprecision of feeling, Undisciplined squadrons of emotions."

Turning now to idiomatic phrases that include the words care and caring, we find there are many. Feeling cared for is certainly one, and there are many others such as care about, cared about, not caring, uncaring, a caring attitude, the caregiver, the cared-for, giving care, doing care, nursing care, health care, legal care. The list of idiomatic uses and phrases is long.

I believe that the specific phrase studied, feeling cared for, means something different from "being cared for" or "being cared about." It is quite possible that a person may be in a dependent state due to illness or age (very young or very old) or some other life situation (a dinner guest who is being well hosted or a male graduate student whose wife is working so that he may be in school), and be the recipient of what could be termed care and yet not *feel* cared for. This would seem to be the case when we so often hear people remarking, "[Person's name] did _____ for me, but he [she] doesn't really care about me." The emphasis is often on the "really" in this sentence, "she doesn't *really* care about me," implying that the recipient ends up without any feelings of having received care or caring.

In all such phrases, it seems that the word care must be or is being qualified and that always it is context driven in the sense that the meaning of the phrase is dependent on the context of the situation being described. Perhaps the word care is in some ways hollow or empty of explicit meaning in that it always has to be explained further if we are to understand its meaning.

Finally, the study of these etymological sources did lend support to my original bias that the phrase *feeling cared for* is not easily explained.

Participants' Experiences

The following examples of experiences described by the participants have been divided into several sections based on *who gave care,* according to the participants: family, professionals, friends, and so on. The specific *things they did* are described in the examples themselves and most examples are presented verbatim.

Family.   There were more instances of the participants describing experiences of feeling cared for within their families than of any other kind. Parents, spouses, children, siblings, and grandchildren were all mentioned as family members who gave care. What they gave or did or conveyed was different.

Parents were described as providing childhoods that were full of love, affection, material things. Mothers were mentioned more frequently when participants were describing caring felt during an illness, but otherwise, fathers and mothers were mentioned equally. Three examples of parents providing care that resulted in cared-forness are:

I had an idyllic childhood in a rural area of Massachusetts, with lots of children, seven, counting cousins . . . lots of fresh air and fun . . . with parents who were committed to giving the children a stable, joyful childhood . . . we weren't spoiled, but we were free, free to develop, free to grow, free to climb trees, free to do everything . . . so as I look back on my life, I can see that I was very much loved by my parents. Of course I being the young daughter with two older brothers, I guess I was spoiled. It was all wonderful and it made me very happy and gave me a great sense of self-esteem . . . a real feeling of being cared for . . . there were times when after dinner, my father would be watching television, he'd always either have me sit at his feet or sit on his lap. He always hugged us and kissed us. My mother the same way . . . she used to sew a lot and would copy the latest fashions so I was always in style . . . and that made me feel loved . . .

I grew up in a home where my parents cared a great deal for each other as well as for us children. My father showed his caring primarily by taking care of the responsibilities of providing for his family financially, although he also was affectionate with us. My mother did the main nurturing of the family . . . very well. I had a mother who was an extremely nurturing mother. I mean one, not too much, wonderfully. Just very affectionate and very attentive to emotional and physical needs . . . there's still that sense that if I needed to be tucked in I would never be too old . . . (my mother did) physical measures, the presence,- reliability, consistency. My mother was always the first one to pick me up, you know, at school when I was little. If I was sick and the school nurse called, she was there in five minutes, it was this tremendous trust that I knew that it would always be there. She didn't work, but I don't think that would've changed much, she would've been there. We were always first and we knew it.

I remember many instances of my parents being very caring people . . . both as parents and as good neighbors to people less fortunate than themselves. My father took my mother and three of us youngest children to Germany for three months in the middle of the Depression, perhaps on the assumption that if things got worse, he'd never be able to take us and he wanted us to see our heritage and family.

Other experiences of feeling cared for by parents had to do with times of illness. Three examples of this type of experience are as follows:

The greatest caring I remember was when I was in the third grade I had to have my tonsils out, and I remember being constantly cared for by my mother. I remember lying on the bed in the back bedroom, watching the 7-Up bottle's bubbles go up, you know, in my drink right by my bed. And it was very traumatic for me in the second grade when my mother had to go away to work. She hadn't been a working mother before then. And so it was a great privilege, she was really making a big sacrifice to come home from school, to be away from her job, and to take care of me, watching the bubbles go up . . . and I still sometimes when I'm sick, when I'm sick I nearly always drink soda, like I'm drinking right now . . . and I think that part of me associates soda with being cared for. It's like some kind of nourishment. Dr. Pepper and 7-Up in particular.

Initially I was very fearful . . . [woman describing her experience of being on bedrest for several months to keep from aborting a pregnancy] . . . my mother didn't live real close, but she did take on that real mother-child role again with me, and that felt good . . . I think that lying in bed and waiting for people to take care of me was reminiscent of a childlike experience, it really was. And after I got used to it a little and I acclimated a little bit, I began to enjoy it a little bit. It's so like a luxury on some level. Because no one expected anything of me and at first I missed it, but after I got over the withdrawal of not having this giving that I like to do and need to do for my own confidence and my own sense of well-being . . . it was like a self-indulgent experience that I probably, I thought I may not ever have again . . . even though I did experience the anxiety, there was almost a kind of enjoyment in a certain way, like, almost like, like a childlike way, and of being, of going back to that real secure time, you know, as when Mommy tucked me in, and I still have very, have a lot of association with those times. I had an extremely nurturing mother.

When I broke my foot, I did have people taking care of me. My mom and dad are super people, Mom was over here practically every day, doing things for me, which was kind of nice to a certain extent, though I don't want her to be working hard or whatever . . . that was a physical thing that made it difficult for me to get around and I think it made me a little lazy . . . because you get in the habit of having things done for you. My dad is really terrific, if there's something that's broken . . . he will do anything . . . he's real gentle and he had a lot of love for me.

Spouses were described as a "daily presence, beloved company," and "a spirit that is always with me." Three examples of such descriptions are:

My dear wife took excellent care of me. We were married for 50 years. In fact, it was at a point where all I had to worry about was to provide an income and take care of the manly jobs around the house. Everything else she handled. She cooked my meals, did my laundry, provided me with a well-kept home, and best of all, she was patient and understanding. As a result, I became 100% dependent on her for all my needs. In spite of all this goodness, I must admit, the thought of her "caring" for me never entered my mind. After all, as my wife, she was merely performing her duties. It was not until she passed away that I awakened to the fact that for 50 years she was caring for me and our two boys. Then I really felt cared for, but it was too late.

And now . . . I have an extremely nurturing husband. Extremely! Not necessarily to me emotionally, but in the fulfillment of responsibilities type thing, I mean you see a guy walking kids down the street or pulling them in a wagon, I bet he's my husband . . . he's very attentive to the children, always fulfills his home and family responsibilities and he is as consistent and reliable as you could ever imagine . . . my husband would try to do all kinds of thoughtful things when I was laid up that time during the pregnancy, but it was difficult for him because it was his child also and his wife, but he would bring me nice little thoughtful things, usually food, that was his way of showing caring, bringing me food . . . it was very thoughtful.

I guess the greatest person who had an impact is my fiancé . . . his spirit is always with me and I just feel very cared for, I feel we are very much in tune with each other. We are very much alike and I feel that he has had the greatest influence in the area of caring . . . I met him in graduate school and we get along famously, both of us are somewhat perfectionists so that I can allow him to do certain things and I know that they'll be well done . . . he supports me emotionally, socially, academically . . . we have a real strong bond.

Adult children were described by older people as making them feel cared for by taking them on trips; offering to let them live with them; sending a card; crying with worry when a parent was not home on time (one night the participant had come home late to find her daughter crying because she was so worried that something had happened to her . . . and that made her feel really cared for . . .), sending food; making phone calls, visiting.

Paid-for-Service Persons. Professionals or "paid-for-service care-takers" were the next most frequently mentioned group of persons who gave care. Although the participants were themselves healthy, many of them remembered times of illness as times when people did things that resulted in the feeling of cared-for-ness. Doctors were mentioned twice, once as a person who really listened and once as a person who was really nice:

He doesn't tarry, but he does listen. Whatever you're saying to him, he picks up . . . but if you happen to hit him with something that's out of the ordinary, that demands his attention, he breaks his pace right then and there. He cares. He cares.

He was so nice, I mean it's just incredibly nice . . . you know, he met me in the office, I walked into the waiting room and he was there waiting for me . . . both the doctors in the group are very, very special . . . they're the kind that if you're fully clothed they'll knock on the door before they come in . . . because they feel like you have your dignity and people shouldn't be barging in . . . they care about you as a person, not just a case . . . you're an individual and they want to be supportive in every respect . . . as bad as the hospital doctors and nurses were, they were the opposite . . . maybe partly because they have a better clientele . . . they have sincerity . . . they treat you like an individual.

Nurses were mentioned in four instances and were remembered as instilling faith, checking on the participant in a consistent way, doing little things, and treating the participant like an individual.

This little nurse, she was so wonderful: one minute I was crying and I wasn't ever going to walk again . . . and then when I had to start getting up, I didn't want to get up, I fought it, but I finally got into it. She said I'm going to teach you how to pivot . . . I swear she pulled me through those four days. She was an angel. Everything about her, she was stern, she was going to make me do what she wanted to, but yet she was sympathetic . . . .

I used to look forward to seeing her because when she came in she was enthusiastic, asked a lot of questions, such as "how are you feeling," and she seemed genuinely interested in how you really felt.

The nurse checked on me every day with a phone call at five o'clock to see how I was doing (after cataract surgery).

The nurse did a lot of things to make my very painful delivery easier, such as a backrub, changing my position, held my hand, stayed with me . . . and telling me to take deep breaths . . . I was so impressed by that woman that she would be so concerned and care for me enough to do that . . . and there was a black nurse one time who was absolutely marvelous . . . they had put me on forced labor and I was in agony, I felt like I was lying on a brick road and she came into me, and she said, "I'm going to make you feel better" and she did. She turned down the pitocin and turned me over and she rubbed my back and she did all kinds of things for me that made me feel like a new person and I just felt that was so caring, this woman had such a good heart . . . and I've run into a lot of black nurses who I think are the most loving, if, you know, if that's their nature. . . because of the adversities they live/go through, I think they have more compassion.

Other caretakers, each mentioned once, included a physical therapist, a homemaker, a telephone operator, a police officer, an orderly, a speech therapist, and a priest. Each of these instances described some time when the caregiver made the recipient feel special or provided reassurance or did some tangible favor.

Friends. Friends were the last group of caregivers mentioned by a number of the subjects. Friends were remembered as listening without giving advice, loaning an apartment rent free for a winter when the participant was without a place to live, giving a head-and-neck massage before a difficult dental appointment, bringing food, and doing little things when the participant was sick. Specific examples are:

> *He was one of those types of people who would just think quietly, and walk around when he had a problem and he was the kind of guy you would go to for advice . . . and I had a math problem from evening school that I couldn't solve and so I started to talk to him about it . . . and I realized I couldn't explain the problem to him and he said to me, "You know what your problem was was that you didn't understand what the problem was and you were trying to answer it . . . so when you go home tonight, first thing, forget about everything except one thing. Say, what are they asking? What are they really asking? When you understand what they're really asking, you'll get the answer." And I came home and I think it took me two hours and I solved it. But what it was, was his caring. He listened, and that's it; he was always like that, he would always listen to you, and whatever it was he would tell you what, how to do this thing. Very caring person.*

> *And I said: "Jean, would you give me a massage right before I go to have oral surgery?" I knew I was going to be nervous, but I also felt that nerves are literal things, they're not just emotional feelings, they're literal things and that if my nerve is relaxed, it's going to be less likely to be sticking out there and to be, you know, worried about the oral surgeon's scalpel, or bothered by it. And so she gave me a total head and shoulder massage before I left. I know that she could sense that my breathing was short. And she said to me something that I had really wanted to ask for, because they put you under with anesthesia. I really wanted to ask a friend to come after me and to take me home, but in New York, where no one has cars and everyone is so busy I thought that would be being a big baby. But she said it for me. She said, "Isn't there someone to pick you up at the dentist's office? I have an appointment, so I can't do it, but*

*maybe we can call Gina and she could do it." So she called Gina
and Gina did meet me . . . and see me home.*

Various Other Sources of Care. Two people mentioned support
groups as being caring by being nonjudgmental, accepting. These
groups were described as "providing a type of unconditional love and
a real feeling of trust," and "groups that always are caring . . . I've
been in Alanon and Gamblers Anonymous and they really are caring
groups of people who understand the hard things people go through
in this life."

Two people mentioned animals as offering protection, affection,
attention, things that made the person feel cared for:

*When I am physically sick, my cat will sit right beside me, and kind
of watch me or else he'll sleep right beside me . . . the other
cat . . . when I'm psychically disturbed, he'll come up and lick me
on the neck and look at me and meow . . . that's a feeling of being
cared for . . .*

*Animals give us unconditional love . . . this dog, too, he takes care
of me, don't you pal? He watches over me when strangers come. He's
been with me for nine years.*

Two people mentioned times when neighbors did things for them
and helped therefore in ways that made them feel cared for. Both of
the following examples describe next-door neighbors:

*My husband was doing a lot of crazy things and my neighbors would
really help me out . . . many times by helping make decisions about
how to handle something with him . . . they would feed me, help
with chores if I needed it and help me with decisions . . . never ex-
pecting anything in return . . .*

*Then I had a neighbor, an elderly woman, not that elderly, 60, who
was very functional and real lovely and she was next door, and
her husband worked during the day, so she was thrilled to have
someone to keep her company, she sat with me a good portion of
the day and she taught me to knit, that was her way of caring, she
was there for me.*

Two people mentioned strangers doing very kind things . . . the college employee who made me feel like "I could do it" . . . the hospital roommate who "gave me a card and invited me to church with her on Mother's Day." Two people mentioned acquaintances: one mentioned fellow employees who "gave me a wonderful retirement party," and another mentioned a car dealer who never forgets his name.

One person mentioned God as always caring for her. She described God as:

Caring for me constantly . . . I know every day that He cares for me. I know it, I mean it isn't that I believe it, I know it, I experience it over and over.

Another person mentioned that she feels cared for by herself at times. She described going to a museum and buying a new painting as ways she cares for herself:

I guess the first type of experience where I feel cared for is that I took care of me, like when I sometimes do something special for myself, something special that I like, I really get a feeling of taking care of myself. I enjoy and like art, that's like my avocation and when I can either see by going to museums or if I can purchase something I appreciate, I can then go on and appreciate pieces of art or something for years and something that gives me you know, it just gives me a lot of pleasure . . . a lot of self-caring.

There were eight instances when people described things that make them feel cared for, no matter who does it. Being listened to with time and patience and with no advice given was important to two people. Having little everyday things done for you during an illness was mentioned by two people:

When anybody did anything for me, came and brought me an ice cream cone, brought me a book, brought me a model airplane, that, those were the things . . . I like to be pampered and I think I, you know, it's kind of like what I try to do if somebody in my family is sick. I try to make them comfortable and do for them the things that I'd like to be done . . . I like telephone contact with people, physical things like backrubs, food like ice cream and Pepsi, a little stocked refrigerator right next to my bed . . . a private bathroom.

So part of my fears, as a single person, that I was crying about, was what if I have a serious illness? I have no parents (both are dead). My friendships are good . . . especially now that I'm connected with the church, but I just lamented over and over, part of what I was crying about was that who would care the most? Who would worry with me, that kind of hour-by-hour worrying about whether or not this thing was cancerous or this and that until the biopsy came in . . . what I'm talking about is that morning and evening kind of caring, "How was your day?" "Hi, hello, this is me, I'm sick, could you bring home some soup and some yogurt because that's all I can eat." It's that assumptional kind of caring, you know, assumptional caring when you're really sick is crucial.

Finally, four persons mentioned these four different things: the recognition of a hurt or pain or vulnerability, an extended hug, a smile as a way of recognition, and a hello to an elderly person.

Specific Things Symbolizing Feeling Cared For. During the interviews, I asked the participants if there were any particular things that symbolized to them the experience of feeling cared for. Examples of such things that reminded the subjects of the experience of feeling cared for included a portrait of a young woman, a painting of two young women sitting gracefully outdoors, the poem "Splendor in the Grass," a Mother's Day card that was handmade, an audiotape made by the subject entitled *Love Letters of the 1940s,* an old TV show like *Little House on the Prairie,* and old family photos from the early part of this century. Some of these items are included in the section "Literary and Artistic Sources."

Examples of Not Caring. Examples of not caring were solicited from everyone interviewed. With only two exceptions, all the examples centered around situations in which the person or people from whom one would normally expect caring (medical professionals, parents, spouses, friends, repairmen, emergency medical workers) didn't give it in a way perceived as caring by the recipient.

The examples given about the medical personnel were all blatantly uncaring, if not outright cruel. Following are four such examples:

This was the third time I had called the nurse. And I don't like to take pain medicine but she kept saying that she'd call the doctor and this was the third time I called her and I couldn't stand the pain anymore and I wanted something to happen for me not to feel this. And she, she was pretty well disgusted with me and so she came in this time and she says, "Mr. Z., it's all in your head."

And they were wheeling me down to the operating room; I had appendicitis, and I was in terrible pain, you know, to the point where they felt that I was lucky that the appendix didn't burst. Now this is just the opposite, this is not caring. We went down this hall and I don't know who this guy was, and I knew that he was dressed in the attire of doctors and I was going by, and this is very hard to believe, God's honest truth, the guy, as I went by, he did that to me in my stomach (hit him). And you know, he hit me on the side. I almost went through the ceiling.

The nurses ignored me because they thought I was too demanding (patient was on total bedrest because of a broken pelvis). . . . The staff were letting me "vegetate" . . . they were overburdened and burned out and I was so dependent on them . . . I couldn't move . . . it was worse than horrible . . . I felt like I was being punished . . . you're totally at their mercy . . .

One of the things I remember, and I look back and laugh at it, but when they rolled me in, they said that you couldn't get out of bed. And somehow I knew how to ask for a urinal but I didn't know about, what to do about the bedpan. So it was about a month, I just didn't go to the bathroom, for a month! And luckily, one of the nuns picked up on it and it dawned on somebody I wasn't asking for a bedpan. It was really awfully embarrassing and I felt pretty uncared for!

The examples about families not caring included parents who were alcoholics and unreliable and untrustworthy; parents who "never hugged me and said I love you or you're a nice little girl"; parents who were not affectionate; parents who were overwhelmed with five children; and a mother who spanked and screamed at a child in a store when that child was fascinated with the pretty things in the counter.

This last example was given by a woman who said it had not happened to her, but that she'd seen this happen in a department store:

A mother is running through the department stores at Christmas trying to get her shopping done and under great stress, and the children are gazing in the cosmetic counter where all the pretty ribbons and the tinsel and everything is . . . and the mother came up and spanked the child terribly. She said, "I told you to stay with me!" . . . and the child would be in tears and so forth . . . the child was merely fascinated . . .

Other examples of not caring included a description of a husband who was an alcoholic and who did many destructive things when the wife wanted to end the marriage; a wife who wouldn't teach her husband how to any of the household chores when he retired and wanted to help and to learn in case he ever had to do them (which he did, for she died soon after he retired).

There were two examples of friends who, when asked for help, gave what they wanted to give instead of asking and giving what the person wanted. Two other examples were about repairmen who didn't fix what they were supposed to fix, and people at the scene of an accident who were more trouble than help.

There were two examples of the uncaring experienced when the public around a person is insensitive. One example described a young child who could not afford a Boy Scout uniform and subsequently experienced ridicule from his peers. This same young man later in his life could not afford cotton socks in the summer, and he heard the girls in his office making fun of his wool socks; both experiences left him feeling very hurt and uncared for.

The last example of experienced "un-caring" was from a woman who had always felt very cared for in her home with her family. When she went away to college and was in the adjustment period during the first year, she felt terribly alone and forgotten and awful:

I felt afraid that things would come up that I couldn't do for myself . . . not physical things but more like dealing with things . . . I didn't know whether I was going to make it through school . . . I was looking for other relationships (other than her family), and so what I would say not caring, to me, would be not having relationships and not feeling the strength within myself to feel good alone.

There were numerous other examples given by the participants, but the ones presented were chosen because of their especially meaningful descriptions. They were put into the categories assigned after the theme identification.

Literary and Artistic Sources

In searching for descriptions of feeling cared for in the arts, I asked professional colleagues, friends, family, and participants in the study to suggest any material they knew of that described or depicted what they thought was the experience of feeling cared for. In no particular order and without identifying the person who suggested the work, they are presented now.

A Granite Statue of "The Prodigal Son," by Heinz Warneke.   The statue is located in Washington, D.C., on the grounds of the Washington Cathedral and is a statue showing the prodigal son returned from his wanderings, on his knees at his father's side, being lovingly embraced by the father. The person who suggested this as a symbol of feeling cared for said it was "a wonderful depiction of feeling cared for." The statue, whose reproduction here was not possible due to the difficulty with reproduction of a color photograph, does depict an accepting, loving embrace that is unmistakably symbolic of an attitude of sincere caring of the father for his "prodigal" son.

A Song, "Sweet Child of Mine," by Guns and Roses, 1987.   This song was suggested by a 21-year-old man as one that reminded him of the childhood experience of feeling really cared for.

> *she's got a smile that it seems to me*
> *reminds me of childhood memories*
> *where everything was as fresh as the bright blue sky*
> *now and then when I see her face*
> *it takes me away to that special place*
> *nd if I stared too long I'd probably break down and cry*

whoa . . . sweet child of mine
whoa . . . sweet love of mine

she's got eyes of the bluest skies
and if they thought rain
I'd hate to look into those eyes and see an ounce of pain
her hair reminds me of a warm safe place
where as a child I'd hide
and pray for the thunder and the rain to quietly pass me by

whoa . . . sweet child of mine
whoa . . . sweet love of mine

A Passage from the Book Beloved, by Toni Morrison, 1987. In this passage, Morrison describes one woman feeling cared for by an old friend. The main character, Sethe, has just described to an old friend, Paul D, a terrible beating she'd received at the hands of her former masters. At the time of the abuse, her breasts had been full of milk for her infant daughter whom she had just sent off on her way toward freedom in the company of the child's older brothers. The abusers had emptied her breasts of their milk and beaten her back so badly with a leather strap that the scars now looked like the trunk and branches of a tree, a chokeberry tree.

She opened the oven door and slid the pan of biscuits in. As she raised up from the heat she felt Paul D behind her and his hands under her breasts. She straightened up and knew, but could not feel, that his cheek was pressing into the branches of her chokeberry tree.

Behind her, bending down, his body an arc of kindness, he held her breasts in the palms of his hands. He rubbed his cheek on her back and learned that way her sorrow, the roots of it; its wide trunk and intricate branches. Raising his fingers to the hooks of her dress, he knew without seeing them or hearing any sigh that the tears were coming fast. And when the top of her dress was around her hips and he saw the sculpture her back had become, like the decorative work of an ironsmith too passionate for display, he could think but not say, "Aw, Lord, girl." And he would tolerate no peace until he had touched every ridge and leaf of it with his mouth, none of which Sethe could feel because her back skin had been dead for years. What she knew was that the responsibility for her breasts, at last, was in somebody else's hands.

*Would there be a little space, she wondered, a little time, some
way to hold off eventfulness, to push busyness into the corners of
the room and just stand there a minute or two, naked from shoulder blade to waist, relieved of the weight of her breasts, smelling the
stolen milk again and the pleasure of baking bread? Maybe this one
time she could stop dead still in the middle of a cooking meal—not
even leave the stove—and feel the hurt her back ought to. Trust
things and remember things because the last of the Sweet Home
men was there to catch her if she sank? (pp. 17, 18)*

A Relationship in "The Death of Ivan Ilyich," by Leon Tolstoy,
1967.   The story of the relationship between Ivan and the peasant
boy, Gerasim, is told by Ivan. He describes feeling very much cared
for by the boy who ministered to him without denying his illness as
so many others in his life did.

*Gerasim had acted as a sick nurse to the dying man and Ivan Ilyich
had been particularly fond of him . . . Gerasim smiled again and
turned to leave, but Ivan Ilyich felt so good with him there that he
was reluctant to have him go . . . It seemed to Ivan Ilyich that he
felt better when Gerasim lifted his legs up . . . Gerasim did everything easily, willingly, simply, and with a goodness of heart that
moved Ivan Ilyich. Health, strength, and vitality in other people of-
fended Ivan Ilyich, whereas Gerasim's strength and vitality had a
soothing effect on him . . . Gerasim was the only one who understood and pitied him . . . . It was a comfort to him when Gerasim
sat with him sometimes the whole night through, holding his legs,
refusing to go to bed, saying, Don't worry, Ivan Ilyich, I'll get a good
sleep later on; or when he suddenly addressed him in the familiar
form and said, It would be a different thing if you weren't so sick,
but as it is, why shouldn't I do a little extra work . . . He wanted to
be caressed, kissed, cried over, as sick children are caressed and
comforted. There was something approaching this in his relationship with Gerasim, and so the relationship was a comfort to him.
(pp. 99-104)*

Two Privately Owned Prints by Unknown Painters.   These
prints were hanging in the homes of two of the participants and
were described by them as artistic things that depicted for them the

experience of feeling cared for. Both prints were in soft pastel colors and did not reproduce well in black and white. One showed two young girls sitting in lovely long pastel dresses in some field next to a woods. They are apparently simply enjoying the out-of-doors, not necessarily talking or reading, but just sitting quietly.

The second picture was also of a young woman, but in this picture, one sees the woman only from her waist up and she has her hands folded beneath her chin and is looking wistfully into the distance. Again, the colors of her clothes are pastel and she has on a large graceful, wispy looking wide-brimmed hat.

The Twenty-Third Psalm. This was suggested by an adult as representing the passage in the Bible the best describes caring. The psalm represented for this person the experience of feeling cared for as promised by God. The words of the psalm describe the numerous ways in which God cares for the psalmist.

> *The Lord is my shepherd, I shall not want. He maketh me to lie down in green pastures: he leadeth me beside the still waters. He restoreth my soul: he leadeth me in the paths of righteousness for his name's sake. Yea, though I walk through the valley of the shadow of death, I will fear no evil: for thou art with me; thy rod and thy staff they comfort me. Thou preparest a table before me in the presence of mine enemies; thou annointest my head with oil; my cup runneth over. Surely goodness and mercy shall follow me all the days of my life: and I will dwell in the house of the Lord forever.*

Excerpts from "Ode: Intimations of Immortality from Recollections of Early Childhood, William Wordsworth by T. Hitchinson, 1967. This poem was mentioned by one participant as being of great comfort to her when she was in a particularly stressful period in her life. She said she would read the poem and feel warm and cared for; she especially liked the following sections:

> *Our birth is but a sleep and a forgetting:*
> *The Soul that rises with us, our life's Star,*
>   *Hath had elsewhere its setting,*
>   *And cometh from afar:*
>   *Not in entire forgetfulness,*

And not in utter nakedness,
But trailing clouds of glory do we come
From God, who is our home.
Heaven lies about us in our infancy!
. . . .

What though the radiance which was
           once so bright
Be now for ever taken from my sight,
      Though nothing can bring back the
           hour
Of splendour in the grass, of glory in the
           flower;
      We will grieve not, rather find
      Strength in what remains behind;
      In the primal sympathy
      Which having been must ever be;
      In the soothing thoughts that spring
      Out of human suffering;
      In the faith that looks through death,
In years that bring the philosophic mind.

A Relationship in the novel To Kill a Mockingbird, by Harper Lee, 1960.   This story describes, among other things, the relationship between two children and the reclusive, possibly retarded or mentally ill man next door, Boo Radley. At the end of the book, Boo Radley saves the children from being killed by a man who believed the children's father had disgraced his name. The following passage captures the experience of feeling cared for as told by Scout, the little girl, as she remembers the things Boo Radley had done for her and her brother over the years.

> *Boo and I walked up the steps to the porch. His fingers found the front doorknob. He gently released my hand, opened the door, went inside, and shut the door behind him. I never saw him again.*
> *Neighbors bring food with death and flowers with sickness and little things in between. Boo was our neighbor. He gave us two soap dolls, a broken watch and chain, a pair of good-luck pennies, and*

our lives. But neighbors give in return. We never put back into the tree what we took out of it: we had given him nothing, and it made me sad. (p. 281)

PHENOMENOLOGICAL REFLECTION

According to van Manen (1984, pp. 59–63), phenomenological reflection involves two major steps: conducting thematic analysis and then determining essential themes. The first step of conducting thematic analysis has four parts:

1. Uncovering thematic aspects in life–world descriptions.
2. Isolating thematic statements.
3. Composing linguistic transformations.
4. Gleaning thematic descriptions from artistic sources.

I began this process while validating that the transcriptions of the tape-recorded interviews were accurate. This chore provided me with the opportunity to really listen to the material, a chance for a "first reflection." No attempt was made to spell out any themes per se during this first listening. The intent was simply to validate the transcriptions and to let the material "in" to my mind. Several days passed between the initial reading of the transcripts and the time when I highlighted, line by line, all the material that seemed to be describing experiences of feeling cared for. This material was then outlined and taken back to the participants for their feedback on accuracy.

Once sure that the experiences were accurate portrayals of moments when the participants felt cared for, thematic analysis began on what had turned out to be 53 descriptions of experiences of feeling cared for and 18 experiences of not feeling cared for. It quickly became apparent that each situation described had two component parts; who did the caring and what they did. The actual feelings involved were very rarely elucidated, even when I probed for them in follow-up interviews. It was as if the feeling was cared-for-ness, and acceptable synonyms were few: good, accepted, warm, secure, loved.

The following themes were identified; in order of frequency mentioned, with the most often mentioned being listed first, participants said their needs are met by:

- Family members.
- Persons paid for services.
- Friends.
- Strangers.
- Animals.
- God.
- Support groups.
- Acquaintances.
- Self.

After much reflection and thought about how to group the identified needs, it occurred to me that the specific needs mentioned by the participants all fit into Maslow's hierarchy of needs (1970, pp. 35–47). The hierarchy was not what was important or even relevant here, but the comprehensiveness and the simplicity of the categories used by Maslow. While others' ways of categorizing needs could have been used (Orem, Watson), Maslow's categories did seem the simplest and the easiest for laypersons to understand. Thus, the essential themes relative to specific needs would be:

- Basic physiological needs.
- Safety and security needs.
- Belongingness and love needs.
- Self-esteem needs.
- Self-actualization needs.

With this reflective analysis in mind, I began the phenomenological writing of the experience of feeling cared for. What emerged over time was the material presented in the next section entitled "Phenomenological Writing about the Experience of Feeling Cared For." I then went back to the participants with two things for them to consider: the preceding list of themes discovered within the interviews, the literature and art, and the resultant phenomenological writing about the experience of feeling cared for. Participants agreed that the themes and the final description did accurately describe the experience, as did the ten colleagues I polled.

PHENOMENOLOGICAL WRITING ABOUT THE EXPERIENCE OF FEELING CARED FOR

The experience of feeling cared for is most often remembered as something that happens within a person's family. Earliest memories are of parents who cared for the child in very concrete ways, providing affection, love, food, clothing, a home, attention to the child when ill, and a general sense of security and safety. Persons whose parents could not provide these things describe difficult childhoods and adult experiences that often include more times of not feeling cared for than feeling cared for. Other family members—spouses, children, and siblings—often do things that make people feel cared for. These things include numerous and varied favors or kindnesses, financial and physical security, and beloved companionship.

People outside families who do things that make people feel cared for include persons paid for services (doctors, nurses, physical therapists, police officers, salespersons, etc.), friends, neighbors, and acquaintances. The things these people do include everything from treating people when ill with dignity and respect, and really listening without advising, to simply remembering the person's name. Perhaps because we expect caring behaviors from people we pay for services, these are the people most often and most heatedly mentioned in descriptions of situations that leave people feeling not cared for.

Others who are cited as providing opportunities for people to feel cared for include animals, God, and the self. Such examples are very specific to individuals and their life-styles and values.

The experience of feeling cared for is one in which needs are met without the recipient having to ask. It is an experience that leaves the person feeling secure, loved, and good. The mother with her baby at her breast is probably the purest example of a person offering another the experience of feeling cared for, and perhaps because this is such an early experience and occurs well before the child can speak or conceptualize, the experience of feeling cared for is forever difficult to capture in words for most people.

One participant of this study shared the following experience. His words seem to capture the essence of this human experience, and the story is this:

I recall an experience that occurred when I was a youngster, 10 years of age, as if it happened only yesterday. That year the winter was extremely cold. Although the monetary situation of my parents was poor, the adverse weather forced my mother to purchase a woolen cap for me. It sure felt most comfortable on my head that morning when I walked in bitter cold to school which was about a mile from home.

Back in those days we did not have lockers or even a cloakroom in our school to hang up our belongings. Instead there was a rack in back of the classroom. I placed my jacket and the newly purchased cap amongst the large accumulation of clothing, for we did have over 40 children in the class.

That afternoon, when the time came to leave, the children, including me, made our usual beeline to the back of the room to don our winter gear, but lo and behold, I found my jacket but not my cap. I could not believe it. It was not there. In panic I waited in the classroom for a time in the hope that someone would come back with the cap when they discovered the error, but no such luck.

I was terribly frightened. Even at that early age, I realized the great sacrifice my mother made to obtain the cap for me and I went and lost it on the first day. I was certain that I would be punished for my carelessness even though it really was not my fault.

I stood outside the school building in that zero weather, afraid to go home. A small child frightens easily. So, there I was, shivering and crying when the priest of our church parish noticed my plight and asked what was my problem. I explained the difficulty and my fear of facing my mother.

This person really was a man of God. He took my hand and we walked across the street into a general store. He told me to select a cap that nearly matched the one I lost. As this incident occurred 60 years ago, I do not remember the color of the cap I lost but I do recall that what I picked was almost identical to the one I lost (even my mother never noticed any difference). The priest then paid for it and I was on my way home, somewhat late but greatly relieved.

Now that is what I classify as "caring" that leaves one with a lasting impression. I shall never forget this good deed as long as I live! (Ziober, 1989)

REFLECTION ON THE MEANING OF THE FINDINGS

I began this study in an attempt to increase understanding about the experience of feeling cared for, with the hope of adding fresh insight to the ongoing quest for knowledge about the concepts of care and caring. A method of study was sought that would allow me to, as Maxine Greene put it, "break with the cotton wool, of habit, of mere routine, of automatism to seek alternative ways of being, to look for openings" (1988, p. 2). The method also had to be one that would allow for the collection of personal stories with all the embellishments that these might include. Phenomenology offered such a method, and yet the philosophy of phenomenology is such that although commonalities can be posited, there may be no such thing as a single meaning. There are instead, different vantage points, different stories, different voices. To identify one final statement or "phenomenological writing" about the experience of feeling cared for as the best and truest description of the essence or meaning of the experience may be to nullify the phenomenological premise that the meaning of an experience is embedded in the life of the person being studied.

Having made this qualifier, of sorts, it is true nonetheless that I did identify themes in the participants' interviews, was able to identify specific groups of persons who were remembered as caregivers and was able to classify the needs being met as all fitting into Maslow's needs categories. Furthermore, a written statement was arrived at that seemed to capture in a few paragraphs the core or the essence of the experience of feeling cared for. But does this statement *really* capture the experience? The participants and ten non-participants said it did, in a general way. With one exception though, everyone questioned believed that the story at the end of the phenomenological writing did a better job of explaining the experience than the paragraphs before it. They seemed to believe that the specific example was more descriptive of the reality of the lived experience than the summative paragraphs, even though they did all agree that the entire statement did include somewhere in it, accurate references to their own life experiences. It seemed as if the participants really believed that their own individual stories should have been included in the writing if the writing was to be really inclusive.

All of this points to the fact that while some generalizations can be made about the experience of feeling cared for, the best way to understand the experience may be to read or hear about it from an individual who has had it. Pat Benner (1984) believed in the importance of this kind of understanding when she chose to use exemplars to teach about nursing practice, letting the words of the individual nurses speak to the reader rather than her (Benner's) analysis of those words. Consequently, her books are filled with verbatim descriptions of real-life experiences from the nurses she has interviewed.

Another way to describe such an experience as cared-for-ness in a way that would enhance one's ability to understand it would be to write about it in some imaginative way (poetry, fiction). Watson used such a method to "explain" when she wrote a poem about Australian Aborigines' experiences with loss and caring (1985, pp. 94–100). She had previously written the usual phenomenological writing about the experience and on impulse, decided to also try writing about the experience in poetry. Both formats are available for study in her work (1985, pp. 87–100), and it is striking to compare the two and note the much greater richness of description in the poem than in the paragraph written "phenomenologically." In summary, Noddings, Gilligan, Benner, and Watson all invite us to consider care and caring issues as they are embedded in human experience, with all the complexities and all the hard-to-quantify relationships.

To return to this study, it was found that a phenomenon that could be termed a feeling-cared-for phenomenon or "cared-for-ness" was an entity, a reality, in the lives of the participants. The participants did describe many experiences of feeling cared for, but I believe that all the experiences shared by them were best understood in the context of their lives. Is it phenomenologically correct to arrive at one general statement about such experiences? Surely it must be acknowledged that in writing one final phenomenological description, the researcher is using an experiential shorthand of sorts. The danger lies in the possibility that in attempting to simplify phenomena so that they are more easily shared with others, the result can be so watered down that it loses real meaning.

If there is meaning in the findings of this study, it probably lies in the data itself and not so much in the phenomenological writing about the data. It lies in the examples cited by the participants, who often struggled to recollect and then reconstruct the experience for me. The examples often seemed to them to be so simple and so personal that they wondered aloud how their experiences could help anyone else. Well, they do help. They help us to realize how very important parents and family are in the experience of feeling cared for. They help us to realize that talking about caring and feelings is very difficult to do and consequently very time consuming. They help us to know that feeling cared for is a result of being protected, being provided for, being listened to, being hugged and held, being loved, being remembered . . . the list goes on, and the specifics are always embedded in the lives of the people telling the story. If indeed we want to understand the experience of feeling cared for, we must ask people for their own stories, their own felt needs, their own ways of being made to feel physically and psychologically safe, secure, loved, respected, and recognized as individuals.

The process of conducting this study helped me to know first hand the truth of Joan Tronto's statement:

Attentive to the place of caring both in concrete daily experience and in our patterns of moral thought, we might be better prepared to forge a society in which care can flourish. (1987, p. 663)

Tronto is cautioning us to pay attention to caring if we hope to increase its presence in our lives. Furthermore, Benner (1984) supports the idea that caring must always be studied in context:

Caring is embedded in personal and cultural meanings and commitments. Therefore the strategies for studying it must take into account meanings and commitments. (1984, p. 171)

So the meaning of the findings lie as much in what is not said in the final phenomenological writing as in what is said. It tells us that feeling cared for occurs in families, among friends, is facilitated by paid-for-service people and others, and is felt most strongly when needs are met without the recipient asking that they be. But it ends with an example from the life of one man that reminds us the real meaning lies in the lived experience.

IMPORTANCE AND RELEVANCE OF THE STUDY FOR NURSING

This study set out to uncover the meaning of the experience of feeling cared for in the lived experiences of healthy adults. The findings showed that feeling cared for meant having one's needs met, preferably without asking, and preferably, by one's family. The findings also showed that lived experiences of feeling cared for are best understood within the context of a person's lived life. For nursing, this points to the need to know more about how to identify needs without having to ask directly and how to see that families know how important their involvement is to their family members.

In the area of clinical practice, nurses need to be encouraged to identify ways in which their clients can be made to feel cared for. It is an oversimplification to think that a nurse can go up or down Maslow's hierarchy of needs or Watson's categories, or anyone else's, for that matter, except as a way of checking to see that all categories of needs have been considered. This would be a process that participants in this study might say is irrelevant. The important factor is not to meet all needs, but to meet those the patient believes are important at any given time.

How does a nurse know what needs a patient wants met? A number of studies have been done and reported in the literature review that identify behaviors resulting in cared-for-ness as reported by specific kinds of patients (women in labor, myocardial infarction patients, home-care patients). These are certainly important studies and their findings are being reported in the literature of those specialities. These studies give us very good ideas about the kinds of needs these patients have and the behaviors related to those needs that are perceived as caring.

However, the very best way to identify the needs that deserve caring attention would seem to be to learn to become more involved with our patients and their own stories. We must learn ways of understanding just what an illness or a treatment regime means in the life of a patient, and these are things that we can only learn by becoming involved in their lives as they are lived, not as they are lived while in the hospital or the illness system. Benner and Wrubel write so eloquently of this need to get to know the patient's story, what the illness interrupted and how the patient understands his own "situated possibilities" (1989, p. 16). If we can understand the lived life of a given patient, we can then deduce what that person's needs are likely to be. Better still, we could encourage the family to identify those needs that are likely to be present and to find ways to meet them. According to the findings of this study, families have a better chance of providing the patient with an experience of feeling cared for than any other persons or groups.

Nursing education could be doing some specific things to increase the likelihood of nurses practicing in ways that result in cared-for-ness. Since the best way to identify areas that need caring attention is to get to know the patient's story and get more, not less, involved, we must find ways of teaching this ability to "get involved." We certainly need to continue to stress the importance of careful listening, careful attending to "the other." But we also owe it to our students and ourselves to take the time to see or read or hear as many human examples of lived experiences of whatever phenomenon we are studying as possible. More time spent in studying the humanities, those time-tested subjects that concern themselves with the lives of human beings rather than their biological systems, would increase our abilities to appreciate the subtle and the major differences in the lives of human beings. Students could probably learn more about the roles that caring plays in the lives of human beings from guided reading and studying of the literature of Dickens, Tennyson, Dickinson, Tolstoy, Morrison, and many others than from reading the same number of research studies about the subject. Furthermore, studying the humanities paves the way for seeing more rather than fewer of the possibilities inherent in any situation, as a person is forced into contact with people different from him- or herself when reading.

When this study began, I had no idea that one of the major recommendations would be that we need more of the humanities in our nursing curriculums. Humanities often take more time and attention than other more practical courses, but acting in ways that result in persons feeling cared for also takes more time than doing more practical things. Learning to be patient and quietly attentive to the world in which we find ourselves, whether with patients or ourselves, would go a long way toward enabling us to really see the meaning and the needs in patients' lives and to then empower the right people (family, friends, or professionals) to do those things that would result in the patient feeling cared for. More valuing of the humanities and their focus on the concerns of individual human beings throughout time would be one clear way of demonstrating that human beings are the subject of nursing, not their medical conditions.

Research in nursing needs to continue to focus on the study of care and ways of caring. It is encouraging to note that more research is now being done on the topic of care and that some journals are publishing such works, but more needs to be done. This study pointed up several areas that deserve more attention and research.

Society has traditionally assigned the role of caretaker to women. The participants in this study, however, did not mention mothers more than fathers, or women more than men. Was this a significant finding that flies in the face of prior assumptions about caregivers? If so, what does it mean and how might it change the way we perceive mothering or caregivers?

The study revealed the importance of families to the experience of cared-for-ness, and more work needs to be done to investigate this aspect of caring. How can we encourage our clients' families to seek ways to provide experiences of cared-for-ness for their family member who is ill? When there is no family available, does caring delivered by professionals suffice? Can professionals ever provide care that can equal that given by a family member? The more we can learn about what it is that families do, the more we will know how to simulate them and how to support them.

In reviewing the findings and the meanings of the findings of this study, readers might ask, so what? Just because the experience of feeling cared for can be described by individual healthy adults, does that mean that nurses can now provide care that results in patients feeling cared for? And even if nurses could provide such care, would patients' loneliness decrease? Would knowing about cared-for-ness help us prevent childhood psychopathology induced by parents who don't care or who cannot care? What if everyone did feel cared for? Would we have a world of more happiness, more community, less illness? Is caring and the experience of caring necessary for survival?

More and more people seem to be saying yes—caring is essential. The mother whose quote was shared at the beginning of the study said, "We need caring so desperately" (Reilly, 1978, p. v). Noddings (1984, p. 12) said:

> *If we can understand how complex and intricate, indeed how subjective, caring is, we shall perhaps be better equipped to meet the conflicts and pains it sometimes induces. Then, too, we may come to understand at least in part how it is that, in a country that spends billions on caretaking of various sorts, we hear the complaint, "Nobody cares."*

Tronto (1987, p. 663) encourages us to be more attentive to the place of caring in our lives if we are ever to forge a society in which care and human beings can flourish.

If, in fact, we are to say that we value human beings and that we care for them as nurses, then we must continue to find ways to understand what this means in the reality of the lives of our patients and in our own lives. This study has shown that feeling cared for is a real human phenomenon. It cannot be learned about apart from the life of the human being experiencing it. It is usually the result of one person's increased attention to and involvement in the life of another. It is a phenomenon that requires time and human involvement. It should be primary to nursing.

REFERENCES

Ainsworth, M. (1966). *Deprivation of maternal care: A reassessment of its effects.* Vol. II. New York: Schoken Books.

Benner, P. (1984). *From novice to expert: Excellence and power in clinical nursing practice.* Menlo Park, CA: Addison-Wesley.

Benner, P., & Wrubel, J. (1989). *The primacy of caring: Stress and coping in health and illness.* New York: Addison-Wesley.

Constantino, R. (1988). The meaning of caring in nursing. In Wang, J., Simoni, P., & Nath, C. (Eds.), *Proceedings of the West Virginia Nurses'*

Association, 1988 Research Symposium: Power through excellence (pp. 73-79).

Eliot, T. S. (1943). *Four quartets.* New York: Harcourt Brace Jovanovich.

Gaylin, W. (1976). *Caring.* New York: Avon.

Gilligan, C. (1982). *In a different voice: Psychological theory and women's development.* Cambridge, MA: Harvard University Press.

Greene, M. (1988). *The dialectic of freedom.* New York: Teachers College Press.

Griffin, A. P. (1983). A philosophical analysis of caring in nursing. *Journal of Advanced Nursing, 8,* 289-295.

Guns N' Roses (1987). Sweet child of mine. (Cassette Recording, *Appetite for Destruction*). Warner Brothers Records.

Harlow, H. F. (1959). Love in infant monkeys. *Scientific American, 200,* 68-74.

Hillman, J., & Von Franz, M. (1979). *Lectures on Jung's Typology.* Irving, TX: Spring Publications.

Hitchinson, T. (1967) (Ed.). *Wordsworth: Poetical works.* New York: Oxford University Press.

The Holy Bible, King James Version (1946). New York: Collins.

Lee, H. (1960). *To kill a mockingbird.* New York: Warner.

Leininger, M. (1981). *Caring: An essential human need.* Thorofare, NJ: Slack.

Leininger, M. (1984). *Caring: The essence of nursing and health.* Thorofare, NJ: Slack.

Leininger, M. (Ed.) (1985). *Qualitative research methods in nursing.* Orlando, FL: Grune and Stratton.

Maslow, A. (1970). *Motivation and Personality.* (2nd ed.). New York: Harper & Row.

May, R. (1969). *Love and will.* New York: Norton.

Mayeroff, M. (1971). *On caring.* New York: Harper & Row.

Morrison, T. (1987). *Beloved.* New York: Knopf.

Moustakas, C. (1961). *Loneliness.* Englewood Cliffs, NJ: Prentice-Hall.

Munhall, P., & Oiler, C. (1986). *Nursing research: A qualitative perspective.* Norwalk, CT: Appleton-Century-Crofts.

Noddings, N. (1984). *Caring: A feminine approach to ethics and moral education.* Los Angeles: University of California Press.

Reilly, D. (1978). *Teaching and evaluating the affective domain in nursing programs.* New York: Slack.

Shipley, J. (1945). *Dictionary of word origins.* New York: Philosophical Library.

Tolstoy, L. (1967). The death of Ivan Ilyich. In *Great short works of Leo Tolstoy*. New York: Harper & Row.

Tronto, J. (1987). Beyond gender difference to a theory of care. *Signs, 12*, 644-663.

van Manen, M. (1984). Practicing phenomenological writing. *Phenomenology and Pedagogy, 2*, 36-69.

Watson, J. (1979). *Nursing: The philosophy and science of care*. Boston: Little, Brown.

Watson, J. (1985). *Nursing: Human science and human care: A theory of nursing*. Norwalk, CT: Appleton-Century-Crofts.

Watson, J. (1987). Nursing on the caring edge: Metaphorical vignettes. *Advances in Nursing Science, 10*, 10-18.

Ziober, J. (1989). Personal communication.

APPENDIX A

Table of Comparative Approaches

Comparative Approaches[*]

van Kaam (1969)

1. Preliminary Considerations
   - Identification of phenomena to be studied.
2. Identification of the Research Question Evoked by the Experience
   - What are the necessary and sufficient constituents of this feeling or experience? What does the existence of this feeling or experience indicate concerning the nature of the human being?
3. Awareness Phase of Explication
   - During this phase, the phenomenon's component parts emerge.
   - This is achieved by explanations of the phenomenon gathered in writing from the subjects.
4. Scientific Explication
   - Data are ranked and classified according to the frequency of occurrence.

[*] Developed by Brenda Blanchette (1993); adapted from Omery (1983).

- This ranking is verified by expert judges.
- Number of categories is then reduced to eliminate overlapping, vagueness, or intricate categories.
- These categories are again verified by expert judges.
- Hypotheses are developed to theoretically explain the categories.
- These hypotheses are tested on a new sample to determine if any new categories emerge.
- This process is continued until no new categories emerge.

5. Final Identification and Description Data
   - Complete description of phenomenon.
     - Requires large sample.
     - Data collected is in writing.
     - Utilizes participants as well as experts for confirmation of findings.

Giorgi (1970)

1. Description of Experience
   - Small sample is chosen to be interviewed. Lengthy interviews that may take several sessions.
2. Data Analysis
   - Read entire description (notes of transcriber) to get a sense of the whole.
   - Read again more slowly, identifying constituents not by frequency of occurrence, but by intuitive judgment by the researcher.
   - Eliminate redundancies in the units, clarify the meanings of the remaining units by relating them to each other and the whole.
   - Transform constituents from concrete language (in the subject's words) to the language of the interested science (such as nursing).
   - Integrate the insights into a description. This is then communicated to other researchers for confirmation and criticism.
     - Smaller sample size.

- More concerned with "the whole."
- Utilizes only experts for confirmation of findings.

Colazzi (1978)

1. All subjects' oral or written descriptions are read in order to obtain a feel for the whole.
2. Significant statements and phrases pertaining directly to the phenomenon are extracted.
3. Meanings are formulated from these significant statements and phrases.
4. Meanings are clustered into themes.
5. Results are integrated into an exhaustive description of the phenomenon.
6. Researcher returns to participants with description for validation. Any additional new data is incorporated into the fundamental structure of the experience.

van Manen (1984)

1. Turning to the Nature of the Lived Experience
   - Turning to a phenomenon that seriously interests us and commits us to the world.
2. Existential Investigation
   - Investigating experience as we live it rather than as we conceptualize it.
3. Phenomenological Reflection
   - Reflecting on the essential themes that characterize the phenomenon.
4. Phenomenological Writing
   - Describes the phenomenon through the art of writing and rewriting.
     - Utilizes researcher's personal experience.
     - The study of an experience as one lives it, not as one conceptualizes it.
     - Utilizes descriptions located in literature and art.

Qualitative Research Proposals:
Form in the Service of Substance

This Appendix suggests a format or proposal that would be congruent for qualitative research design in its broad sense.

Because acceptance or rejection may be based on following prescribed outlines, the significance of such outlines or materials needs to be addressed by the nursing scientific community.

The aim is to provide the forms necessary to communicate the substance. Also, this format has been acceptable in universities and students have found it is most helpful. It is still not phenomenological as might be the Outline in Appendix D, but it is a useful educational way to go about learning this different approach. Unfortunately, critical substance gives way to form. The processes of approval, acceptance, and funding are philosophically and politically influenced by the formats available to us to frame these inquiries. Theory building research needs, however, distinctive formats to maintain the aim and integrity of the particular method.

A CASE EXAMPLE

Upon reviewing a qualitative dissertation proposal that was written according to the quantitative research proposal outline for a specific institution, many compromises and inconsistencies were found: The first chapter of the proposal spelled out the "required theoretical framework" and a "specific nursing theory" that the study would use. The proposal stated that a specific nursing theory "will provide the theoretical perspective of the lived experience: of the phenomenon under study." The researcher then provided a full description of the preselected framework, and how she would be validating or testing the theory with her study. The second chapter—on methodology— then contained a quotation from Omery (1983) saying that "to ensure that the phenomenon is being investigated as it truly appears or is experienced, the researcher must approach the phenomenon with no preselected theoretical framework" (p. 50). This placed the researcher in a contradictory position. The material (i.e. the proposal format she had used) was not reflective of her method: the substance and form were not philosophically or methodologically congruent.

THE NEED FOR SPECIFIC GUIDELINES

It has become apparent that specific guidelines for proposals for qualitative research methods are necessary to maintain the integrity of the research method. Broadly speaking, qualitative research is concerned with discovery and, to the extent possible, a theoretical. In contrast, quantitative research is more concerned with theory validation and confirmation. The latter starts with a deductive approach to hypothesis testing or theory testing (Leininger, 1985; Munhall & Oiler, 1986). Because the two approaches rest on different philosophical premises and methodological rules and processes, a proposal for a qualitative research design should differ substantively in syntax, logic, and process. In other words, specific guidelines for qualitative research proposals will facilitate nurse researchers in articulating specifically the aims and methods of qualitative studies.

What is suggested here is a proposal format for qualitative research. Emphasis is made that form is in the service of substance; whatever it may be, the form is quite secondary to the substance of the study. However, from the historical perspective at this time in nursing research, qualitative proposals, in addition to being primarily attuned to substance, must also provide:

1. Education about, and description of, the method, from its aim to its outcome.
2. Justification for using this method.
3. Translation of any unfamiliar language into words that will help the reader understand the method better.

Provision for these processes are within the following guidelines.

RESEARCHING THE PROPOSAL

The outline that is to be presented here has been in use in a major doctoral institution for 7 years and in many other educational settings. The evaluation of the students and the response of faculty have resulted in an ongoing process of continual revisions. However, the integrity of the proposals and reports has been gratifying, and the author looks forward to more refinement.

PROPOSAL FOR QUALITATIVE RESEARCH METHODS

Introduction: Aim of the Study

The aim of the study involves the inquiry into a *phenomenon of interest*. What the researcher needs to communicate in this introduction is the *perceived justification for studying* this phenomenon. Since a method for discovery is being used, the fundamental aim of the study will be to find out "What is it like?" "What is this?" or "What is going on here?" Other questions, such as "What is the nature of this experience?" or questions probing cultural patterns or processes associated with certain social interactions, are broad types of research questions that may be asked. A *specific problem statement would then be premature,* as would be a research question with identified variables, since the research is designed to explore the phenomenon of interest without preconceived notions or hypotheses about problems or predicted variables.

The phenomenon should be *discussed within the specific context* in which the researcher desires to study it (e.g., what is going on in a

Table A–1
Proposal for Qualitative Research Methods

1. Introduction: Aim of the Study	a. Phenomenon of interest b. Perceived justification for studying phenomenon c. Phenomenon discussed within specific context (e.g., a lived experience, a culture, a human response) d. Assumptions, biases, experiences, intuitions, perceptions related to belief that inquiry into phenomenon is important e. Qualitative research method chosen with justification of its potential f. Relevance to nursing
2. Evolution of Study	a. Rationale b. Historical context c. Experiential context
3. Method of Inquiry—General	a. Introduction to specific method b. Rationale for choosing method: philosophical and theoretical substantiation projected c. Outcome of method d. Background of method e. Sources (individuals) whose methods will be followed f. General steps or procedures of the method. Plan for literature review g. Translation of concepts and terms
4. Method of Inquiry—Applied	a. Aim b. Sample c. Setting d. Gaining access e. General steps f. Human subject considerations: informed consent, entry, departure, confidentiality, secrets, process consent—when and if situation should change g. Strengths and limitations h. Anticipated timetable i. Actual feasibility of study—Are access and cost possible?
5. Appendixes	a. Supporting documents b. Consent forms c. Communication
6. References	

"special" type of nursing home? What is it like to feel healthy at a particular developmental phase, and why is this relevant to nursing?).

Exploring nursing homes in a qualitative inquiry would give us a description of the culture, patterns, and processes associated with that particular context. Problems may be discovered, areas where nursing intervention is needed may become evident, and a theoretical base for hypothesis formation could be developed from the field of origin. A *brief review* of the qualitative method chosen by the researcher, along with its appropriate outcome, should be included in the introduction section. The researcher's own experiences, intuitions, assumptions, and preconceptions can be included here as well, with reference to their further articulation in Sections 1 and 3 (see Table A-1).

The overall purpose of this introduction is to orient the researcher and reader to the phenomenon of inquiry and the broad design. It should convince the reader of *the importance of discovery and exploration* vis-à-vis a specific qualitative design. The researcher also demonstrates in the introduction how the aim of the study has important implications and relevance for nursing. The researcher demonstrates clearly the substance of the study.

Evolution of the Study

In this section, the researcher places the study in the *context from which it has originated.* Here readers of quantitative research proposals are most accustomed to come to understand, from a thorough literature review that supports the study, why the researcher is studying the phenomenon. In qualitative designs, the literature review is more often postponed in the interest of maintaining a clear vision, one that is not theory ladened or biased. Experience, to the extent possible, is seen afresh. Nursing conceptual models and frameworks, if used this early in the study, might also selectively frame, or give direction to, the data. Like the literature review, they, too, are brought in after data collection, when the researcher wishes to establish how the results of the study broaden, or are compatible with, a particular theory or nursing conceptual model.

In a description of the evolution of the study, the researcher again provides a rationale for the study and can support this rationale with a *historical context* (that which the researcher already knows about) and an *experiential context* (that which is in the researcher's own experience). Here the researcher should speak of personal experience, often a starting point in exploratory studies. For example, "I came to realize that almost all the patients in this nursing home exhibited some signs of depression" and then go on in a descriptive, narrative way.

The overall purpose of this section is to describe the evolution of the *researcher's origin of interests,* and to place the study into its *historical and experiential context.*

The Method of Inquiry—General

This is a critical component of the qualitative research proposal because of the needs to both educate the readers who may not be familiar with the method, and translate arcane terminology into a language accessible to the average reader. If, for instance, the researcher is going to use a phenomenological design, be it that of Van Kaam (1969), Merleau-Ponty (1956), Spiegelberg (1976), or Georgi (1970), or van Manen (1984), the processes need to be discussed in the clearest terms. This is where both *education and translation come into play.* Phenomenological terminology is not readily understood and is often not within the experience of most nurse researchers or readers of research.

Words or expressions such as "the study of essences," "a caring attunement," "embodiment," "primacy of perception," and "reviewing contacts with original experience" need therefore be clearly translated into simpler terms. Statements such as "phenomenology begins in silence" or "we become the question" are not always comprehensible to the reader. The researcher can actually profit from a thorough translation, since it often requires of him or her to confront the concepts to be explained with his or her own experience, thereby resulting in a deepened understanding of these concepts.

In grounded theory, basic social processes, core variables, and theoretical codes are also phrases that need translation. When describing the method, it is therefore in the researcher's best interest to translate the conceptual language of that method into familiar, understandable terms.

This section is primarily concerned with the process of the *specific qualitative method itself,* whereas the next section will be devoted to applying the method to the researcher's study. In years to come, this section may be no longer necessary; at the present time, however, this overview of the methods is critical to the understanding by faculty, grant reviewers, and students of how the researcher is going to use a given method, and *how that method "works."* The researcher thus introduces in readily readable language the specific method, *gives the rationale for choosing the method,* and describes the philosophical underpinnings. The background of the method, as well as the outcome and importance of this type of method need to be emphasized (i.e., what the method will produce for nursing, and why is it important). If, for instance, the identification of basic social processes within settings helps us create nursing interventions, it should be highlighted. If a phenomenological baseline is critical to nursing theory development, it needs be underscored. An overview of the process, including a brief description of what each step entails, should be provided. Here, for example, if the phenomenological inquiry included bracketing, intuiting, analyzing, and describing, each of these steps would be described (Oiler, 1982).

The Method of Inquiry—Applied

It would be helpful for the researcher to repeat here *the aim of the study,* and then to show *how* the actual application of the method will *accomplish the aim.* The researcher will then go through the procedure as discussed in the preceding section, but without the details of the specific study. In grounded theory, for example, the researcher will describe how the processes of memoing, sorting, saturation, literature review, and conceptualization are to be carried out within specific parameters of this particular study.

With most qualitative methods, the sample needs to be selected according to preestablished guidelines. The sample size may not be as important as in quantitative studies, however. If interviewing individuals about a particular phenomenon, the researcher might, for instance, continue the interview process until new information no longer becomes available. When repetition or redundancy appears in the data gathered either from a single individual or a group, the saturation point may have been reached—no new information is to be obtained at that time.

In this section, the researcher communicates the characteristics of, as well as the *rationale* for, the selection process. Suggestions for *selecting participants* or *sites* to be used in qualitative research studies can be found in texts that deal with particular methods.

The *setting* and how the researcher is going to *gain access* must be described. The phenomenon of study guides the selection of both the setting and the sample. The departure from the quantitative format consists of describing in a systematic way how the researcher will be going about obtaining experiential descriptions from subjects.

In keeping with the generalized expectations of readers and reviewers, this section should also include the *details,* format, and procedure of the planned *interviews,* the *participants' observations,* the *way data will be stored,* and the *particulars* of *reliability* and *validity* of the method used. A researcher contemplating qualitative research needs to clearly differentiate how the concepts of reliability and validity are addressed from the particular perspective. A good text on the specific method will provide this information, which, again, needs to be translated.* In *Reliability and Validity in Qualitative Research* (Kirk & Millers, 1986) for example, the authors distinguish between three kinds of reliability—quixotic, diachronic, and synchronic (see also Sandelowski, 1986). In contrast to such self-explanatory quantitative terms as construct validity or interrater reliability, those types of reliability must be explained and translated. The qualitative researcher has indeed a challenging task, not only presenting a proposal, but also translating and teaching a method.

Human subject consideration should be included in this section as well. In addition to traditional concerns, the qualitative nurse researcher needs to address the handling of entry, departure, secrets, interviews, observations, and information, from the perspective of protecting individual rights. A suggestion for process consent where reviewing and/or renegotiating the informed consent is made from the perspective of the dynamic quality of fieldwork or serial interviewing (Munhall, 1988).

---

* Within this text are other means to evaluate qualitative research (see Chapter 11).

Plans for the dissemination of findings should also be included. In qualitative studies as part of the validity process, findings are often discussed with the participants. Additionally, the researcher may want to project that the findings will be reported in a dissertation, or a research report to a granting agency, to nursing audiences and journals, or to interdisciplinary journals.

A discussion of the strengths and limitations of the study should be attempted. The relevance to nursing and the strength of the particular method should be reiterated for emphasis. *Why* this particular research interest lends itself to a qualitative study can be restated here, as a strength. While we cannot ignore limitations, the usual reference to sample size, generalizability, or probability should not be listed as limitations since they do not hold the same meaning for qualitative research methods. It is also unnecessary to state that the researcher is a limitation, having little familiarity with the method. That has little to do with the method chosen, whether qualitative or quantitative; if it is the first study the researcher has done, who is to say why it may not be the best!

Appendixes

This section is for the most part similar to quantitative research methods, and includes communications, consent forms, human subject approval, and other supporting documents.

References

These are listed according to style.

REPORTING QUALITATIVE RESEARCH STUDIES

When the qualitative study is completed, the researcher will then be ready to write the findings of the inquiry. The proposal, which was written mostly in the future tense as a plan, is now written in the past tense as a report of activities that have transpired. The first three sections (Introduction: Aim of the Study, Evolution of the Study, The Method of Inquiry—General) can remain roughly the

Table A–2
Outline for Reporting for Qualitative Research Methods

1. Aim of the Study	a. Same as proposal. More breadth b. Include now outline of remaining report
2. Evolution of Study	a. Same as proposal b. More breadth and depth
3. Method of Inquiry— General	a. Same as proposal but more specific
4. Method of Inquiry— Applied	
	a. Findings are discussed according to the method. Example: In grounded theory method, the aim is generation of theoretical constructs. In this section, researcher would have findings from the process of: Memoing Theoretical sampling Sorting Saturation Review of literature The theory
5. Findings of the Inquiry	b. With the ethnographic method, findings may be reported in a smooth, flowing description narrative. The aim of the narrative is to portray the full context, to the extent possible, that was discovered by exploring pieces of reality and/or experience. Review of other sources, literature, art, films, etc. c. With phenomenology guiding the method, the findings will be reported differently. An example might include: Description of experiential themes Essences of experience Description of relationships among essences Review of other sources (literature, art, films . . .)
6. Reflections on the Findings	a. Meanings and understandings b. Implications of the study (for whom) c. Relevance of the study (for whom). Integrate: With preconceptions and ideas as discussed in the introduction With existing literature and practice in the area of study With the utilization of the method d. Significance and substance e. Importance to nursing f. Suggestions for future inquiries
7. Appendixes	Dissertation proposals and reports would include all necessary appendixes (e.g., consent letters, tables)
8. References	

same, shortening or lengthening the content depending on the projected audience. The fourth section (The Method of Inquiry—Applied) becomes very specific to the study.

The Method of Inquiry—Applied

In this section, the researcher describes *specifically* how the method was used in *accomplishing the aim* of the study. If the researcher was utilizing the grounded theory method, then the details of data gathering need to be provided: how the researcher coded the field notes; used memos, did theoretical sampling, sorting, and saturation; reviewed the literature, and so on. This section can be subdivided so as to include the literature review after the observations and interviews of data collection are completed. Oftentimes with qualitative research methods, the literature review is considered part of the data collection. The researcher may, for instance, present the interviews, the participants' observations activities, and then a literature review, in that order. Other sources of data to be collected about any given phenomenon through a qualitative lens might include art, films, documentaries, poetry, and other aesthetic forms that express the lived experience and/or culture.

Again, the sample, setting, human subject consideration, reliability, and validity need to be fully discussed specifically as they have occurred in the researcher's utilization of the qualitative method.

Findings of the Inquiry

According to the method, this section will often be reported in a narrative style, to portray to the fullest extent possible, the experience and observations that the researcher has—depending on the method—thematically analyzed, developed tentative theoretical suppositions, and/or synthesized into a descriptive narrative of a specific culture. Diagrams could be used to enhance the narrative, but for the most part this section is "writing." It may be phenomenological writing, writing the theory, or writing the report about the specific culture or subculture. The writer, through words, is articulating findings, and while they are his or her findings, they faithfully reflect the narrative and the portrait of the subjects.

Reflection on the Findings

In this section, the researcher discusses the *meaning of the findings.* What are the *understandings gleaned* from the findings, and what are the possible implications? This section should also bring the inquiry together as a whole, including a comparison and discussion of the findings with the preconceptions and ideas as discussed in Section 1. Attention should be called to the context of the study as the researcher reflects on the findings. Existing literature on the phenomenon also needs to be discussed. Reflections on the method and its outcome should be included along with suggestions for future inquiries. Questions should also be raised.

Highlighted in this section is the importance and relevance of the study for nursing. What is the significance of the discovery of the meaning of a specific experience or a new descriptive theory or a description of a culture to nursing?

Appendixes

References

Provide as in proposal, as well as any additions.

ABSTRACT

Table A–3
Call for Abstracts; Qualitative Research Methods; Titles

1. Aim of the Study	a. Phenomenon of interest b. Relevance for nursing
2. Evolution of Study	Rational, experiential, and historical contents
3. Method of Inquiry—General	a. Brief overview of purpose of method b. Basic steps c. Suggestions for future inquiries
4. Method of Inquiry—Applied	Brief overview of specific steps: sample, interviews, setting, procedures, consent, data analysis
5. Findings of Study	Brief synopsis of findings of study
6. Reflections on the Findings	a. Brief synopsis on the meanings, understandings, and possible implications of the study b. Significance and substance briefly discussed

To be helpful to nurse researchers, planners of research conferences often provide a format for submitting research abstracts. This can be enormously helpful, to the extent that the abstract then is ready to be photostated! The same problems that prompted this effort are often encountered, however: absence of problem statement, of hypothesis, and of statistics, as the format calls for.

Table A–3 is offered as an alternative, and follows the proposal outline as well as the outline for reporting findings (Tables A–1 and A–2).

CONCLUSION

The overall goal with methods of qualitative research is to achieve accurate portrayals, authentic descriptions that enable understanding and valid representation of the meaning of being human, being through an entity. An important consideration for the scientific adequacy of the study is to remain as close as feasible to the philosophical underpinnings and aims of the method. To enhance the substance of the study, rather than manipulate the substance into a different form, a distinctive format in the proposal and report need to be utilized.

Placing qualitative research into quantitative research proposals is like trying to hammer the proverbial round peg into a square hole. Nurse researchers who use qualitative methods find themselves judged poorly because their study cannot be communicated clearly within the traditional research format. I have suggested here a form that will give way to substance. And substance should be what nursing research is all about in the first place.

APPENDIX C

Postmodern Proposal Outline

PHENOMENOLOGICAL PROPOSAL TO RESEARCH

1. Origin of Interest in Phenomenon
2. Discovering a Need for the Study
3. Evaluating Responses to Your Proposed Study
4. Commitment to Listen to Others
5. Interviews and Existential Investigation

PHENOMENOLOGICAL REPORT OF RESEARCH

Phenomenological Research as Writing—the telling of the story of being in a specific experience.

Appendix: Review of Approach Used.

APPENDIX D

Example of Postmodern Outline
Phenomenological Inquiry and Method

Cathy Appleton (1993)
Acting Director, Graduate Program in Nursing
Florida Atlantic University

*T*he methodological structure of human science research explicated by van Manen (1990)* was employed to understand what caring is like for women. Van Manen asserts that hermeneutic phenomenological research is a dynamic interplay among six research activities:

1. Turning to a phenomenon of serious interest and commitment.
2. Investigating the phenomenon as it is lived, rather than as it is theorized or conceptualized.
3. Reflecting on the essential themes that characterize the phenomenon.

* References not included here.

This appendix is an example of brevity, in a good sense, of description of "method." What is important in studies from this perspective is what follows the description and interpretation of the experience.

4. Writing and rewriting to describe the phenomenon as it is present in the lived experience.
5. Sustaining a pedagogical relation to the phenomenon.
6. Balancing the research context by considering parts and whole (pp. 30–31).

As methodology, phenomenology aims to get at the nature of the meaning of every day experience. Consequently, phenomenological inquiry seeks a deeper understanding of a particular phenomenon by researching lived experience.

The phenomenon of this study is central to how women experience their lives. Personally as a woman, and professionally as a nurse, caring has always been pivotal to my experience. As a researcher, I explored the meaning of the art of nursing and discovered that caring emerged as integral to the practice of nursing when it is art (Appleton, 1991; 1993). When I researched the experience of caring in nursing education, central to student competence and intellectual development is the experience of caring for and about students on the part of the faculty (Appleton, 1990). Consequently, my commitment to know what caring is like for women comes from and is grounded in this personal, professional context.

In publicizing this study, I printed announcements and informed people by word of mouth. Twelve women responded and consented to participate in tape-recorded interviews. I asked each participant, "What is caring like in your experience as a woman?" The interviews lasted approximately 90 to 120 minutes and the tapes were transcribed into text.

Through reading and rereading the texts, and reflecting on the descriptions of caring as these women described it, a process of analysis transpired that explicated what constitutes the nature of caring in women's experience. Thinking deeply about each woman's narrative description of caring and the entire narrative descriptions of all these women assisted me to know the essential themes that emerged as the work of helping; caring on both sides: living the conflict; finding out what matter is in life: taking the risk; incredibly good people: they read of God; and empowering caring in our lives: a mission.

The chapter was organized, thematically, around the essential themes of the phenomenon after initially interpreting the nature of the phenomenon. Context was provided by writing existential or weaving the phenomenological description with existential themes of temporality, spatiality, corporeality, and communality.

"Bringing to speech" women's experience of caring occurred through writing and rewriting (van Manen, 1990, p. 32). By maintaining an orientation to the research question, I engaged in what van Manen (1984) refers to as a "dialectical going back and forth" among the levels of questioning (p. 68). This activity sensitizes the researcher to the language. In an effort to preserve the language of these women, I varied the examples throughout the chapter. In addition, I provided a transcendental form to women's experience of caring by offering literary expression of the phenomenon.

The study of human experience, what it means or the nature of experience as it is lived, is the concern of the phenomenologist— who as a researcher investigates experience as it is, rather than as it is conceptualized. Van Manen (1990) suggests the following questions be asked of the entire phenomenological research study: "Is the study properly grounded in a laying open of the question? Are the current forms of knowledge examined for what they may contribute to the question? Has it been shown how some of these knowledge forms (theories, concepts) are glosses that overlay our understanding of the phenomenon?" (p. 34). I'll let you be the judge.

Study with appendix to appear in *In Women's Experience* (Munhall, 1994) NLN.

APPENDIX E

Example of Description of Perspectives
The Phenomenological Approach

Robin Parker (1992)

Phenomenology as a research methodology concerns itself with gaining access to the outer world (life-world) from the inside of human experience (consciousness). This is accomplished through structured reflection leading to transcendental subjectivity (unmediated intuition) of the meaning of experience through the enrichment of existential (being-in-the-world) and hermeneutic (interpretive) thought (Wagner, 1983).*

Phenomenologists speak of going back "to the things themselves," to begin with phenomena and the experiences, not theories, in an attempt to move science away from positivism and reductionist views of the world (Cohen, 1987, p. 31).

---

* References not included here.

Appendices F and G are examples of what Section Three of the Outline (Appendix B) would be about. Additionally the reader is provided here with a brief historical overview of phenomenology, in both appendices.

"Intersubjectivity, the belief in the existence of others who share a common world, is important to the phenomenological tradition" (Cohen, 1987, p. 31). With regard to this study, it is the belief of this researcher that parents of ADHD children share a common experience during their parenting, regardless of the fact that each of these parents is involved with a different child.

This chapter will present an introduction to the phenomenological method, the rationale for method selection, an overview of the history of phenomenology, Merleau-Ponty's philosophy and Max van Manen's (1983) phenomenological approach to inquiry and thematic analysis.

The natural science and phenomenological perspectives are grounded in different, competing epistemological foundations and paradigms. An epistemological foundation is a branch of philosophy that deals with knowledge, and how we come to know about the world as we experience it. A paradigm is a philosophy, or belief or worldview (Munhall, 1986). Opposing central tenets underlie both the natural science and phenomenological perspectives.

First is the fact that each perspective has a different view of men or women in the world (Morse, 1991). The natural science tradition has a reductionist approach, whereas the phenomenological approach is a holistic orientation to the study of the individual. Second, the natural sciences treat meaning as "facts," whereas the phenomenological tradition maintains that "meaning is contextually constructed as an intersubjective phenomenon" (Morse, 1991, p. 31). Human beings create meaning by interacting with one another. Third, these opposing perspectives' aims are different. The natural sciences seek causal explanations, predictions, and control, whereas the phenomenological approach seeks understanding and interpretation (Munhall, 1988). Fourth, the natural sciences are characterized by deductive reasoning, objectivity, and statistical techniques. In contrast, phenomenology is characterized by inductive reasoning, subjectivity, discovery, and description (Ray, 1985).

The word "phenomenon" in phenomenology refers to objects, events, situations, and circumstances as they appear to a participant in original perception, prior to any interpretation. "Experience," on the other hand, refers to living through an event, situation, or circumstance. The aim of phenomenology is to disclose lived experience, but it is recognized that the closest one can come is to disclosed perception (Oiler, 1981).

The term "perception" has a distinctive meaning in phenomenology and warrants elaboration. Perception is the original awareness of what one lives through in experience. It is in the nature of being human, however, that one interprets her or his awareness. Meaning emerges from the inextricable interrelationship of person-world as a person gives meaning to experiences. The reality of an experience cannot be known apart from a person's experience and interpretation of it. It is important in phenomenology that an understanding of the concepts of experience, perception, and meanings be explicated and clarified.

Since phenomenological methods can be classified as a type of qualitative methodology, they share many similarities with all qualitative methods. Specific differences in this methodology do exist, however. One such difference is the requisite of phenomenology that no preconceived notions, expectations, or frameworks be present or guide the researchers as they gather and analyze the data (Omery, 1983). Second, the phenomenological method makes no assumptions. It does not deny that such things as process might be discovered, but phenomenology does not assume that processes exist before they are described (Wilson, 1989). Third, with the phenomenological method, the researcher approaches the participant and the experience with an open mind, accepting whatever data are given. Phenomenology accepts all experiences as valid sources of knowledge for the participants living the experience. Each experience communicated to the researcher is viewed as valid (Ray, 1987). Fourth, the philosophical basis for this methodology is distinct from other qualitative approaches. This philosophical basis originates with an existential phenomenological view, emphasizing a person as unique, possessing potential and experiencing opportunity for change (Appleton, 1990).

RATIONALE FOR METHOD SELECTION

The phenomenon of the meaning of parenting a child with ADHD lacks both investigation and description in nursing literature. An understanding of this phenomenon of human experience has failed to be adequately elucidated using qualitative methods of inquiry. What one believes to be parenting an ADHD child may not in fact be that experience. Gaining an understanding of this parenting experience is the aim of phenomenological inquiry.

Phenomenology, as a method, seeks to describe and unfold the phenomenon of parenting an ADHD child before the eyes of the researcher and reader, so that the essence of what it means for these parents to parent these special children can be experienced and understood, if only briefly.

PHILOSOPHICAL UNDERPINNINGS OF THIS STUDY

Paterson and Zderad (1976) view nursing as an existential human experience of being and doing with another. According to Paterson and Zderad (1976):

> *Phenomenology involves an openness to nursing phenomena, a spirit of receptivity, a readiness for surprise, and the courage to experience the unknown. (p. 76)*

The act of caring increases the humanness of both patient and nurse. The phenomenological approach can be advocated as the most appropriate for studying the richness and complexity of nursing phenomena.   ˏ

Ray (1992) states, for nurses phenomenology offers a means by which the lived experience of the "life-world" or human phenomena (mental, social, and historical) of the nurses and persons to whom they are responsible can be studied and understood. She states:

> *Phenomenology as a philosophy and a method is a fundamental way through which the nurse clinician or researcher at the beginning of an enterprise secures an absolute foundation for herself. This absolute foundation is the cumulative consciousness for her/ his life-world made explicit by the rigorous process of structured*

reflection which informs show she/he views and experiences the
ever changing world of immediate experience. (p. 56)

It is Ray's belief that one must know and understand the self first
before entering into the life-world of another. For nurses, phenomenology can offer a means by which a nurse can constantly discover and rediscover her/his awareness of the world. Ray supports
nursing's pursuit of the humanistic elements of nursing care by discovering the meaning of caring for individuals, families, and groups.
She asks, if certain humanistic attributes—for example, empathy,
compassion, comfort, trust, support, and protection have been identified as caring phenomena, what meaning do they have for clients?
Ray states rigorous efforts toward identification of meaning are
needed in nursing. According to Ray (1985):

The meaning of a client's reality through the phenomenological ap-
proach will reveal to the nurse the qualities of each individual's ex-
perience, which subsequently will provide a more comprehensive
understanding of the nature of nursing itself. (p. 85)

Oiler (1982) states that "phenomenology is a philosophy, an approach, and a method. Possessed by a reverence for experience, it
conforms to nursing valuing" (p. 178). She goes on to say the phenomenological approach is appropriate because "the nursing profession emphasizing a reverence for clients' experiences, is concerned
with the quality of life, and the quality of the nurse-patient relationship" (p. 180).

Munhall (1988) states that phenomenological studies are needed
in current theory formation and reformation to determine which researcher biases have influenced worldviews and as a result have
helped establish norms and standards that may be inappropriately
generalized. A qualitative perspective then, according to Munhall
(1988):

becomes essential from the philosophical perspective of nursing not
only as a research design but also for actual implementation of a
holistic, empathic, individualized delivery of nursing care. (p. 27)

OUTCOME OF USING
PHENOMENOLOGICAL METHOD

By utilizing the phenomenological method of inquiry and analysis as described by Max van Manen (1984), it is the researcher's belief that a description and increased understanding of what it means to parent a child with ADHD will evolve. This description will be developed from the parent's experience. The outcome of this process will enable the researcher to capture the phenomena of study by uncovering the central themes of parenting a child with attention-deficit hyperactivity disorder.

HISTORICAL OVERVIEW OF PHENOMENOLOGY

Phenomenology is a branch of philosophy which can be divided into three phases: Preparatory, German, and French (Cohen, 1987). Phenomenology's primary historian Herbert Spiegelberg (1960) researched and wrote about the historical evolution of phenomenology using the word "movement" as a means of expressing his belief that this is not a stationary philosophy (Cohen, 1987, p. 31). The fact is, the phenomenological philosophy has transformed and evolved with each different philosopher, and within each of the three phases (Cohen, 1987). A brief overview of the three phases and the significant contributions of philosophers: Frank Brentano, Carl Strumpf, Edmund Husserl, Martin Heidegger, Jean-Paul Sartre, and Maurice Merleau-Ponty will be presented.

This researcher has been influenced most by the philosophy of Merleau-Ponty and the specific approach to Max van Manen (1984) as published in the journal *Phenomenology and Pedagogy.*

In the Preparatory phase, during the last half of the nineteenth century, Frank Brentano (1838–1917), a philosopher, first wrote about phenomenology as a method of inquiry. Brentano is credited with two major contributions that are important to present-day phenomenology. The first was his discussion of the value of "inner perception," which is an awareness of our own psychic phenomena, as opposed to unreliable introspection. The second was the fact that he was the first philosopher to discuss the concept "intentionality," which implies the inseparable connectedness of the human being to the world (van Manen, 1990). Intentionality would be a concept basic to all later phenomenological analysis (Cohen, 1987).

The second philosopher whose work helped evolve the Preparatory phase was Carl Strumpf (1848-1936). One of Strumpf's most significant contributions to the phenomenological movement was his position that the method could be studied with the rigor of experimental and scientific techniques (Spiegelberg, 1978). "Strumpf never believed in dissecting the world at the price of destroying the connections" (Spiegelberg, 1978, p. 60). Strumpf's belief that the essence of experience should not be sacrificed by examining the relative component part of the experience has carried through many of the present-day phenomenological movements.

In summary, the Preparatory phase provided philosophers and scholars such as Brentano and Strumpf with the opportunity to describe the phenomenon (behavior) before testing the behaviors with a traditional scientific method. This was an effort to enhance the nature of psychology.

Edmund Husserl (1859-1938) and Martin Heidegger (1889-1976) dominated the German Phase of the Phenomenological Movement. Husserl was and is considered to be the central figure and primary philosopher of phenomenology (Cohen, 1987). Husserl brought forth the belief that the study of philosophy should have a new humanism versus only "rigor" (Ray, 1992, p. 83). He became disenchanted with the scientific position of positivism-empirism, that is, the facts alone gave the final truth. Instead, Husserl became the first philosopher to propose the use of phenomenology as a creative attempt to apprehend meaning through the study of human experience (Appleton, 1990). Subjectivity began to dominate this philosophy and was the source of all objectivities (Cohen, 1987).

Husserl placed a vital emphasis on the concept "essences" (Cohen, 1987). The term "essence" derives from the Greek "ousia," which means the true being of a thing, the inner essential nature of a thing. The essence is that which makes something what it is (without which it would not be what it is); it is that which makes a thing what it is rather than its being or becoming something else (van Manen, 1990).

Another important aspect of Husserl's philosophy was "phenomenological intuiting" (Cohen, 1987). Spiegelberg (1960) pointed out that
this term is one of many in phenomenology that is difficult to translate into English. Phenomenological intuiting is a direct grasping of
the essential structure of phenomena as they appear in the consciousness (van Manen, 1984). Additionally, Husserl's specific how a
philosopher can recover by phenomenological reduction (structured
reflection), the ability to describe with scientific exactness the life of
consciousness in its original encounter with the world (Ray, 1985, p.
83). Husserl demonstrated how phenomenology, in a rigorously scientific manner, could attempt to explain meaning.

Two major concepts were noted by Cohen (1987) within
Husserl's work. Out of Husserl's work arose the concepts "intersubjectivity" and "life-world" (Levenswelt), the world of lived experiences. Intersubjectivity is what the human science researcher
needs the other (the participant) to develop, in order for the dialogic relation with the phenomenon to occur, thus validating the
phenomenon as described (van Manen, 1990). In this respect, researchers who share this common world, as in the case of this researcher, are required to "bracket" their identification with the
participants' experience if they are to be able to study the phenomenon. In phenomenological studies to this day, this methodological requirement is an essential technique if the results are to be
considered reliable (Oiler, 1981). This technique of "bracketing"
will be used throughout this study.

The life-world is the second concept in the phenomenological
movement credited to Husserl (Cohen, 1987). The life-world is the
world of lived every day experiences. We often fail to notice much
of our every day experiences. We often fail to notice much of our
every day experience because it has become so commonplace to us.
We simply take it for granted. Phenomenological study can help us
to really see that which surrounds us with renewed awareness (Cohen, 1987). Attention is given to the concept of the lived world of
the study's participant(s) as well as the researcher in present-day
phenomenology. The reliability of the study is enhanced with the
explication of the researcher's lived world and the subsequent
bracketing of the experience (Munhall, 1988). This researcher's

world was described in Chapter II within the historical and experiential context of this study.

Heidegger was the second influential philosopher in the German phase. The most universal concept of Heidegger's hermeneutic phenomenology is "Being" (1962). Heidegger uses "Being" as a fundamental term for this ontological analytic, rather than using it to describe an entity or ultimate ground. "Being is always the Being of an entity" (p. 29), and so to ask for the Being of something is to inquire into the nature of meaning of that phenomenon under study. Van Manen (1990) stated, "Being" is a fundamental term of the human science research process itself. Human beings exist, act, or are involved in the world. In other words, the individual participates in cultural, social, and historical contexts of the world and as such is said to "be-in-the-world" (Munhall, 1988).

Phenomenology in Germany came to an end for all practical purposes with World War II and the Nazi years. Before the war, Heidegger became Husserl's assistant. Reportedly, Husserl thought highly of Heidegger and recommended him as his successor. With World War II, Heidegger became intensely involved in the Nazi movement and refused to help Husserl, who was Jewish. Phenomenology moved from Germany to France, after the Nazi takeover (Cohen, 1987).

The French phase of the phenomenological movement recognizes three key philosophers: Gabriel Marcel (1889–1973), Jean-Paul Sartre (1905–1980), and Maurice Merleau-Ponty (1908–1961). Marcel used phenomenology and saw it as a useful introduction to the analysis of "Being." Sartre's goal was to understand because "to understand is to change, to go beyond oneself" (Cohen, 1987, p. 33). Sartre expanded phenomenology as an alternate research method and as a method of inquiry (Spiegelberg, 1976). For Sartre, phenomenological writing became the center of his life. For Merleau-Ponty, phenomenology related to experienced time, space, body, and human relation as we live them. It was Merleau-Ponty who pointed out that the effort to describe human experience as it is lived, is what phenomenology represents. As previously stated, this researcher has been influenced most by the philosophy of Merleau-Ponty and by the specific approach for inquiry and analysis of Max van Manen. The remainder of this chapter will be an overview of Merleau-Ponty's and van Manen's work.

BACKGROUND OF THE METHOD

Merleau-Ponty's Phenomenology

In the 1940s, Maurice Merleau-Ponty began writing about phenomenology; this interest continued until his death at the age of 53 (Spiegelberg, 1984). Merleau-Ponty's themes about phenomenology changed and evolved during the course of his lifetime. Several concepts that are apparent throughout his work emerged. These were the idea of embodiment, the importance of perception or the *primacy* of perception, and the need to focus on lived experience (Merleau-Ponty, 1962). A brief discussion of these themes will follow as they are important to current-day phenomenology.

Merleau-Ponty (1962) became the first French author and philosopher to publish a work with the word "phenomenology" in the title (*Phenomenology of Perception*). In this book, Merleau-Ponty (1962) stated, "We are condemned to meaning" (p. xix). He developed a detailed case for the importance of considering the individual's experience (Cohen, 1987). This direct emphasis on the individual's experience was a rejection of the positivistic conception of science.

According to Munhall and Oiler (1986), Merleau-Ponty has described phenomenology variously as:

> *the study of essences, a transcendental philosophy that questions facts about our world more adequately, and a philosophical stance or position that attempts to describe experience as it is lived without concern for how it came to be the way it was. (p. 48)*

The theme of embodiment according to Munhall and Oiler (1986, p. 52):

> *informs us that consciousness is diffused throughout the body and finds expression through it. We are our bodies. Bodily position in space and time, bodily movement and action shape experience by giving consciousness access to the world. There is in experience, then, a unity of the perceiving subject and the objective world. In experience there are not inner and outer realities.*

For Merleau-Ponty, the idea of embodiment is a way of viewing persons as they are in their world within their body, which is consciously finding expression in feeling, speech, thought, sensing, judging, and so on (Munhall & Oiler, 1986).

Embodiment as described by Merleau-Ponty (1962) is an important idea for two reasons. First, embodiment prevents researchers from being totally objective as we are always being influenced by our own body's situation in the world. Second, the views of the researcher and the participant will differ as each is bound to view the world from his or her own specific stance dependent on that person's own body and own situation in the world.

Primacy of perception is the next theme described. According to Merleau-Ponty (1962, p. 42):

Perception gives one access to experience of the world as it is given prior to any analysis of it. To perceive is to render oneself present to something throughout the body. All the while the thing keeps its place within the horizon of the world.

For Merleau-Ponty, perception is access to the truth, it is also the original mode of conscience. He wrote that people experience the world around them by perception. Perception then becomes a person's truth. Merleau-Ponty believes that perception is a totally unique, individual experience that depends on both the context of the situation and the external stimuli being perceived.

In summary, Munhall and Oiler (1986) state that according to Merleau-Ponty:

Perception is the appearance of phenomena, and the perceived world is reality . . . not to be confused with the truth. As access to truth, perception presents us with evidence of the world, not as it is thought but as it is lived. It is this evidence that is considered to be the foundation of science and knowledge. Beyond this, there is nothing to understand. (p. 57)

The theme of lived experience is the last of Merleau-Ponty's philosophy to be presented in this chapter. For Merleau-Ponty (1962), turning to the phenomena of lived experience means relearning to look at the world by reawakening the basic experience of the world (p. viii). He strongly believed that lived experience was phenomenology's focus.

Van Manen's Approach of Phenomenological Research

While at the University of Alberta, Max van Manen (1984) described the particular phenomenological approach that will be used in this study. Van Manen was strongly influenced by Merleau-Ponty's philosophy and described phenomenological research as a dynamic interplay among four procedural activities. They are:

1. Turning to a phenomenon which seriously interests us and commits us to the world (turning to the nature of lived experience).
2. Investigating experience as we live it rather than as we conceptualize it (existential investigation).
3. Reflecting on the essential themes which characterize the phenomena (phenomenological reflection).
4. Describing the phenomenon through the art of writing and rewriting (phenomenological writing) (1984, pp. 39-44).

The purpose of these procedural activities is to assist the researcher to arrive at a deeper understanding of the nature of meaning of our every day experiences. This increased understanding will ultimately help us become more humanistic and caring as we learn the difficult skill of how to act tactfully in situations based on careful thoughtfulness.

By using van Manen's procedural approach, we not only can learn about lived experience but can gain insight, as van Manen (1984) states:

Phenomenology differs from almost every other science in that it attempts to gain insightful descriptions of the way we experience the world. So phenomenology does not offer us the possibility of effective theory with which we can now explain and/or control the world but rather it offers us the possibility of plausible insight which brings us in more direct contact with the world. (1984, pp. 37-38)

Phenomenology is, according to van Manen (1990), "a philosophy or theory of the unique; it is interested in what is essentially not replaceable" (p. 7). This is in contrast to traditional, experimental research which is largely interested in knowledge that is generalizable. Van Manen also believed that a person could only really begin to understand phenomenology by doing it. This belief originated from Merleau-Ponty. In reading phenomenological research, van Manen states that the significance of the final description is only understood when we understand the amount of work, time, reflection and rewriting that is required in this type of study, "It all seems somewhat absurd until we begin to discern the silence in the writing" (1984, p. 37).

In hermeneutic phenomenological research, as described by van Manen (1984), the first procedural activity involves turning to the nature of lived experience, which involves a thoughtfulness and questioning on a phenomenon of interest that is important to the investigator. The topic of this study comes from both the researcher's personal (family) and professional experiences. There is a passion in my quest for an increased understanding of the meaning of this experience. It is with veneration that I view these parents and children.

In phenomenological research, the researcher *lives* the question by a process of returning to the question or the thing itself (the experience of parenting an ADHD child) until one begins to feel a sense of the nature of the topic being studied. This process is in contraposition to simply stating the question as is the case in other research methods. This researcher also understands that she will function as a "tool" or part of this project as data are filtered through her, read, written, or tape-recorded during this study.

The last part of turning to the nature of lived experience involves explicating assumptions and preunderstandings. With the use of phenomenological inquiry, a common problem is that the researcher has too much information about the phenomenon under study. A researcher must state clearly her or his assumptions prior to and throughout the study so that she or he can bracket them. This researcher stated her assumptions and biases in Chapter I. In addition, the researcher detailed personal experiences and perceptions related to her understanding of this phenomenon to avoid the possibility of researcher bias, which could then interfere with the study's findings.

The second procedural activity will investigate experience as it is lived (existential investigation). This is the data collection or data generation stage. It is here that the researcher will ask, "What is the meaning?" "Can you give me an example?" This researcher will use interviewing by means of open-ended questions and personal journaling to gather information about the lived experience of parenting a child with attention-deficit hyperactivity disorder. Before this process of interviewing begins, this researcher will again explicate any preunderstandings, suppositions and/or assumptions known to her.

Van Manen outlines four steps that should be used to develop an understanding of the phenomenon under study. These are attending to one's personal experience with the subject matter; tracing etymological sources and idiomatic phrases; connecting descriptions from others; and locating experiential descriptions in literature and art.

The first step in the data collection is for the researcher to reflect on personal experiences of parenting an ADHD child. This was done at the beginning and will be done during the process of this study. It is assumed that the researcher will be less likely to interject her own biases into the interviews or analysis by staying close to this process. The second step in the data collection will be the study of the etymology of the words *parent* and *parenting.* This will be done in the library with dictionaries and etymological sources and will be presented in Chapter V. The third step in the data collection is to collect descriptions of the phenomenon of interest from others. Data collection in this study will be from normal, healthy adult volunteers. All interviews will be open-ended and focused on having the participants describe their personal experiences with parenting their ADHD child. The fourth step is locating the experiential description in literature and art. Research participants and colleagues will be asked to share artistic examples of the experience of parenting an ADHD child. The poem by Susan Hughes (1990) which begins this study's description is one such example. In addition, phenomenological studies on the experience of parenting a chronically ill child done by other nurses will be reported in the literature review in Chapter VI.

The third of van Manen's procedural activities, phenomenological reflection, will involve two major steps: conducting thematical analysis and determining essential themes. The final phenomenological description, which will be the end point of this study, will be based on these themes. According to van Manen (1990), "A theme is the experience of focus, the meaning, of point. Themes describe an aspect of the structure of the lived experience" (p. 87). When attempting to uncover thematic aspects, the researcher asks, "What statement(s) or Phrase(s) seem particularly essential or revealing about the phenomenon or experience being described?" (van Manen, 1990, p. 93). The analysis of themes begins with the descriptions of the participants' experiences. From these participant descriptions, the researcher begins to reflect on the lived experience. A clarification of themes begins to evolve as the researcher begins to understand the meaning of the experience as a whole. Developing themes describe an aspect of the structure of the lived experience and allow the researcher to determine meaning from the lived experience data.

The fourth procedural activity, the phenomenological writing, is good if:

> . . . *it reawakens our basic experience of the phenomenon it describes . . . in such a manner that we experience the more foundational grounds of the experience. (1984, p. 65)*

Van Manen (1984) has termed this process of writing as a "poetizing activity" (p. 41). The phenomenological writing should be both an example containing examples as well as a description of this human experience.

The next chapter will present the application of this study's methodological approach (i.e., aim, sample, setting, gaining access, general steps, and human subjects' considerations).

APPENDIX F

Example of
Phenomenological Approach
The Phenomenological Perspective

Maribel Mezquita (1993)

THE MEANS OF INQUIRY

This chapter presents an overview of the phenomenological hermeneutical method and rationale for its selection to guide the study. A historical overview of phenomenology and phenomenology in nursing are illustrated. The specific approach by van Manen and its methodology are also described.

Phenomenology, as a research approach, attempts to study human experience as it is lived (Langer, 1989; Oiler, 1983).* It presents itself as a philosophy and an approach in addition to a research method (Psathas, 1973).

Van Manen (1990) asserts that the aim of phenomenological research is the elucidation of lived experiences through phenomenology descriptions. The accomplishment of such an approach will provide deeper understanding and meaning of our everyday experiences.

* References not included here.

Therefore, the foremost aim of phenomenology is for us to become more human. This belief is congruent with our nurses' goals and values (Munhall, 1992).

The lived experience provides the context from which phenomenological human science begins.

The lived experience is the life-world that involves our immediate, prereflective consciousness of life (Dilthey, 1985). The study of human science is the different approaches and orientations to human research.

Human research entails the diverse aspects of human phenomena such as social, historical, and cognitive. According to Dilthey (1987), human research demands understanding and interpretation. This approach diverges from the scientific research found in the natural sciences based on natural phenomena, consisting of physical, chemical, etc., which require observation and explanation (Edie, 1984).

It is postulated that meaning in our lived experiences is veiled through our involvement in the world or layered with meanings added from our relation of being in the world (van Manen, 1990). Therefore, the phenomenological approach is an attempt to more fully understand and to uncover meaning of our daily experiences as to reveal those aspects which pertain to individual experiences. Such understanding could not be attained with the use of quantitative studies.

Ray (1990) illustrates that phenomenology facilitates a fuller understanding through description, reflection, and directing our awareness of the phenomenon for the purpose of revealing its inherent meanings rather than to observe and explain.

Merleau-Ponty (1964), sustains that we perceive the world through our body, thus perception is our access to human experiences. He adds that the descriptions acquired by phenomenology are those of the perceived world. He clarifies that the descriptions based on individual perceptions are not purely subjective phenomena since there are no subjective phenomena. He argues that objective and subjective are united in being in the world through an inseparable connectedness. For instance, when we think or perceive something, it is not purely a subjective act in our minds, but rather, it is the perception of something in relation to objects in the world through consciousness. This assumption in phenomenology is referred to as intentionality. Intentionality, explained in the works of Husserl, is the most basic human act of translating or interpreting the world of objects and things. Spinelli (1989) suggests that individuals are always conscious of something.

Meaning is found in the intersubjective, which is a subject/participant relationship. Therefore, phenomenology begins in the human experience and our involvement in the world through direct awareness or consciousness. Van Manen (1990) proposes that phenomenological inquiry stems from our own experience or exposure to the phenomenon. In order to understand the structure of something, one has to practice reflection and a certain level of reduction.

Van Manen (1990) explains that the act of reflection is the effort to grasp or to understand the meaning of what we are living through. The data examined in reflection is that of our daily involvement in the world. It is not an interior set of acts, or introspection, which falls in the realm of internal perception.

Reduction is referred to by van Manen as the process of recovering original awareness. In practicing reduction, we assume the attitude of doubt toward the world and what we know of it, including our beliefs, and place them in brackets, or suspend them in order to study the essential structure of experience. In phenomenological description, it is primordial to set aside the natural attitude toward the world. Thus, the end of reduction provides the world that remains after bracketing.

The main principle of phenomenology demands for the researcher to approach the study without any preconceived notions, conceptual frameworks, or expectations and to bracket or to suspend any preunderstandings and assumptions. Although bracketing may be extremely difficult since it may be somewhat impossible to bracket all biases and assumptions, it can be attempted and practiced (Spinelli, 1989).

HISTORICAL OVERVIEW OF PHENOMENOLOGY

Spiegelberg (1965), traced the history of the phenomenological movement and divided it into three phases. The word movement, chosen by him, exemplifies a nonstationary philosophy.

The first phase is referred to as the preparatory phase, in which phenomenology was first introduced as a method of inquiry. Franz Brentano was the forerunner of the phenomenological movement in the last half of the nineteenth century. Carl Strumpf was the founder of experimental phenomenology and first prominent student of Brentano.

Brentano expanded the idea of inner perception versus unreliable introspection. He classified the awareness of psychological phenomena into these related terms, for the purpose of differentiation.

Inner perception was defined as the immediate awareness of our psychological phenomena, including our emotions, while maintaining our attention to the external objects. He credited inner perception as infallible self-evidence. Introspection or self-observation gained his distrust by its unreliability. Central to Brentano's philosophy was the concept of intentionality, which explains that all our psychic experiences refer to objects. For instance, we do not perceive without perceiving something. His concept of intentionality has been slightly modified and has become one of the most fundamental assumptions of phenomenology.

The second phase was the German phase. The prominent scholars dominating phenomenology in the early twentieth century were Edmund Husserl and Martin Heidegger.

Husserl, the student of Brentano, was considered the dominant figure in the movement of phenomenology (Spinelli, 1989). His philosophic radicalism related to the question of becoming or the origin of all knowledge (Speigelberg, 1965). His philosophy was the theory of knowledge, or epistemology. He adopted the notions of subjectivity and searched for his ideal of creating a rigorous science for phenomenology.

Husserl formulated the idea that the life-world, or the everyday world in which we live, and our natural attitude fail to provide immediate accessibility for exploring phenomena. This is due to our taken-for-granted attitude of our natural world; thus, it can only be apprehended through phenomenological study.

Husserl indicated how the process of phenomenological reduction facilitates the practice of reflection. His ideas of reduction have been modified since then and are currently referred to as bracketing out of prejudices.

Martin Heidegger was the second philosopher scholar of the German phase. He was primarily concerned with being and with time (1962). Heidegger was able to refine and converge Husserl's phenomenology with existentialism, constituting what is known today as existential phenomenology. His ideas support that the meanings we assign to our experiences radiate between or are extracted from ourselves and particular situations.

Heidegger's main contribution to the movement was possibly his influence on the French phenomenological movement.

France was receptive to the phenomenological philosophy derived from German leaders. This originated the third or French phase of the movement.

The French philosophers brought preciseness to phenomenology formulating the philosophy and science of existential phenomenology (Ray, 1990). The most prominent scholars were Gabriel Marcel, Jean-Paul Sartre, and Maurice Merleau-Ponty. Phenomenology, as a method of inquiry, was reactivated by Sartre as an alternative to the established scientific research methods (Spiegelberg, 1965). Marcel exposed the concept that phenomenology provided the avenue to explore the ontological or existential questions of being in the world.

Merleau-Ponty (1964) alleges the belief that we are always conscious of something. He clarifies that it is not inner existence but rather it is life. Our bodies provide existence in the world while our awareness and perception are expressed through our consciousness. The unification of body and mind allows for meanings to unfold in relation to our connectedness with the world. Human experience is actualized in the four life-worlds identified by Merleau-Ponty, which are: space, time, body, and human relation.

According to Merleau-Ponty, we bring our individual history and knowledge of the world as a unified experience that constitutes our consciousness. Our way of experiencing the world is through perception.

Thus, the realm of perception shapes individual realities. Phenomenology provides an effort to describe human experience as it is lived.

PHENOMENOLOGY IN NURSING

Paterson and Zderad (1976) were the first to introduce the philosophical notion of phenomenology in nursing in their book *Humanistic Nursing*. Since then, phenomenology has provided a valid research approach in the study of nursing as a human science (Paterson and Zderad, 1976; Leininger, 1985; Ray, 1985; Parse et al., 1985).

The new view that nursing as a human science includes the art and science of human caring is supported by salient nursing leaders (Watson, 1985; Munhall & Oiler, 1986). Nurse researchers and theorists have become disillusioned with the traditional empiricistic or positivistic research methods borrowed from the natural science. The experimental approach presumes the presence of causal relationships through the objectification of subjects. The evidence for determining truth is based on the five senses, which are seeing, hearing, touching, tasting, and smelling (Reeder, 1984). According to this method, important aspects of life such as other modes of awareness are excluded; for example, feelings and intuitions.

As a result, nursing researchers began arguing that human phenomena differed from natural phenomena, requiring interpretation and understanding (Ray, 1990). The method of the phenomenological view integrates all perceptions of human phenomena as real and provides a more comprehensive approach for the study of human science. The act of nursing is defined by Paterson (1978) as, "the intersubjective transactional relation, a dialogue experienced, lived in concert between persons where comfort and nurturance produce mutual human unfolding" (p. 51). In the interrelationship or dialogue between nurse and patient is where meaning surfaces from the depths of experiences.

The search for meaning increases the nurse's understanding of the client's feelings. This transaction influences or changes both the one cared for and the nurse (Watson, 1988). These assumptions enable nurses to be coparticipants in the investigative process.

The science of human caring is the central construct of nursing (Leininger, 1977, 1981). Caring, as defined by Mayeroff (1971), is helping the other to grow and actualize himself or herself. The way nurses can understand human expressions is by descriptions and explications of meaning in the life situations of subjects.

Munhall (1982) asserts that there is an incongruity between nursing philosophy and nursing research.

The core of the nursing philosophy purports the holistic, individualistic view of man. The holistic view grants an integration of man that does not allow the breaking down of his parts for analysis and piecing him back together, typically used by the experimental method (Munhall, 1982).

THE APPROACH OF PHENOMENOLOGY BY VAN MANEN

Van Manen (1990) proclaims that phenomenology is the study of essences. Essences are the nature of phenomena or the essential elements that are required in identifying or differentiating one experience from another. The term essence is best explained by van Manen (1984a) as "a linguistic construction: a description of a phenomenon" (p. 6). It is believed that phenomena have universal essences. These essences can be described through a study of particular instances. For example, the essence or nature of high-risk pregnancy can be accomplished through studying individual or particular mothers' experiences.

The aim of the phenomenological research, according to van Manen, is the quest to become more human as we search to gain insight into the fullness of living.

This human science research method provides the description of the lived experience as it is lived through, known as descriptive phenomenology. Its hermeneutical nature pertains to the domain of interpretation; it is a quest for experiential meaning.

Van Manen (1984) presented an approach to phenomenological inquiry in the early 1980s. His method includes the interplay of four procedural activities. They are the following: (a) turning to the phenomenon which seriously interests us and commits us to the world; (b) investigating experiences as we live them rather than as we conceptualize them; (c) reflecting on the essential themes which characterize the phenomenon; and (d) describing the phenomenon through the art of writing and rewriting (p. 39). Although these activities are presented in sequential order in the outline, they may be performed simultaneously. A copy of the methodological outline is included under Appendix C.

TURNING TO THE NATURE OF LIVED EXPERIENCE

This study was initiated by identifying a phenomenon of interest to be researched. I reflected cautiously on human experiences that could possibly emerge as the topic for the phenomenological study.

The question of what something is "really" like was consequently sparked out of interest from my center of being.

The investigator's preunderstandings, suppositions, and assumptions were explicitly stated in the preceding chapter. They were brought to light for the purpose of avoiding the introduction of biases by the researcher. These biases would interfere with the process of data collection and interpretation of the lived experience.

EXISTENTIAL INVESTIGATION

The process of generating data is performed by the researcher. This active involvement provides a deeper understanding and meaning for the researcher through the exploration of the scope of the lived experience. The researcher should also be sensitive to the way the material is conveyed while remaining open to new possible interpretations. The process of phenomenological investigation attempts to provide understanding of the lived experience from the participant's point of view.

In actuality, the phenomenologist borrows the descriptions of the participant's experiences and reflects on them. Van Manen (1984) explains that this enables the researcher to "an understanding of the deeper meaning or significance of an aspect of human experience, in the context of the whole of human experience" (p. 55).

It is feasible, according to van Manen, for the researcher to have similar experiences and perceptions to those of the participants. Indeed, it is probable that they may have experienced the same phenomenon. This realization may provide the investigator with clues and personal orientation through the avenues of research.

The words that we use to refer to the phenomenon should be traced back to their etymological sources in order to regain their full meaning. The phenomenologist may acquire insight by turning to art, poetry, and literature as rich sources of experiences. The diverse works of art gear the researcher to live experiences vicariously, otherwise not normally experienced. Available phenomenological literature is examined for contextual approaches in an attempt to enable the researcher to reflect more deeply on the phenomenon. The works of other phenomenologists offer a source of dialogue for the researcher.

PHENOMENOLOGICAL REFLECTION

The thematic analysis is the act of reflection by the researcher of the lived experience. This is initiated after the descriptions are obtained. The reflective mode facilitates analysis of the aspects of the structures of the phenomenon. This process allows themes to evolve in a distinctive manner, providing an increased understanding for the researcher. Thus, the meaning of the experience is revealed as a whole. The connection of these themes is required to gain insight and to describe the lived experience.

Van Manen (1984) claims that conceptual formulations or exclusive themes do not capture the lived experience as a whole.

The uncovering of the thematic structures from the narrative descriptions can be facilitated by two approaches. The researcher may read the transcript line by line and determine how each line reveals parts of the phenomenon being described. The second approach is the highlighted approach, which entails the researcher's reading the transcript over and over. As a result, certain aspects of the text are revealed as essential in the experiential description. It is advised by van Manen (1984) that both approaches be used.

The linguistic transformation is a venture into capturing the essence of the themes by the phenomenologist. This process involves the act of writing about their readings and research activities (van Manen, 1984). Paragraphs are developed around the themes, which assist in describing them more distinctly.

The phenomenologist reflects on the phenomenological descriptions with an attempt to recreate experiences. This is referred to as artistic expressions that are not pure imitation of life experiences. Indeed, they represent a transcending of the world of experiences through the act of existential reflection.

The selection of the thematic themes is a fundamental step in the process of thematic analysis. The researcher must determine which themes convey the meaning of the phenomenon as essential. Adversely, some incidental themes may not portray these unique features and must be discarded. In addition, the demand for the themes to fit as a part of the description allows for some themes to be altered or added. Often, the researcher engages in the act of writing and rewriting the text numerous times.

Assistance from the members of the thesis committee can provide insight as to whether the themes and writing are meaningful as part of the fit for the phenomenological description.

PHENOMENOLOGICAL WRITING

Attending to the speaking of language means to be sensitive to the suggestive way language speaks. The attribute for becoming a good listener requires the ability to harmonize with the tonalities of the spoken language, not only with words. It is proposed by van Manen (1984) that phenomenological description is an example of examples. Every example is an interpretation of the original experience although it is not absolute. These interpretations may be added as part of the document, to help illustrate the lived experience for the reader. A powerful phenomenological description will undoubtedly reawaken the primary experience in others who have lived it.

The structuring of the phenomenological description may be organized in several ways although it is beneficial to relate it to the phenomena it is describing. Alternative ways include patterning around the themes; writing analytically; generating the essence of the phenomena by illustrating examples as to how they were determined; weaving existential themes with descriptions; and engaging in a dialogue with another phenomenological author. A combination of these approaches is acceptable according to van Manen (1984). The process of writing and rewriting is expected. It is characterized by back-and-forth careful pondering that allows for the meaning of the experience to emerge. In essence, the methodological process projects as the main goal, to illuminate the meaning of the lived experience and to convey it to readers in a way they can understand (van Manen, 1984).

APPENDIX G

Example of Outline for Course
Nursing Research:
A Phenomenological Perspective

SCHOOL OF NURSING   BARRY UNIVERSITY

COURSE NUMBER & *TITLE*	NUR 6—NURSING RESEARCH: THE PHENOMENOLOGICAL PERSPECTIVE
COURSE CREDIT & *HOURS*	3 credits 45 theory hours
PLACEMENT IN THE *CURRICULUM*	Elective
PRE/COREQUISITES	NUR 602 Nursing Research
FACULTY	Patricia Munhall, ARNP, EdD., Psy.A., FAAN
CATALOG *DESCRIPTION*	Seminar discussions of phenomenological readings to facilitate a beginning understanding of the phenomenological perspective in nursing research. This

course is specifically designed to assist students in comprehending the meaning of the phenomenological perspective for thesis development and practice implications.

CONCEPTUAL FRAMEWORK

The Master of Science in Nursing program is built on seven processes that comprise the practice of nursing: nursing research, change, communication, teaching/learning, administration/management, and professionalism. Research from the phenomenological perspective is critical to all these processes.

COURSE OBJECTIVES

At the completion of this course, the student will be able to:

1. Discuss the phenomenological perspective as a world view for nursing research.
2. Understand the purpose of pursuing research from a phenomenological perspective.
3. Analyze how the phenomenological perspective in research is congruent with nursing's humanistic base.
4. Develop ability to write about experiences from a phenomenological perspective.
5. Interpret meaning from existentially gathered material.
6. Evaluate various approaches of phenomenology to nursing research.
7. Demonstrate how findings from research that are phenomenologically oriented can be implemented into nursing practice.

TOPICAL OUTLINE   Phenomenology as a worldview for research; What is the philosophy of phenomenology about? How does phenomenology contrast with Logical Positivism? What is the purpose of research from a phenomenological perspective for nursing? The Existential Investigation; Finding meaning in everyday experiences; Writing phenomenological texts; Interpretation from a phenomenological perspective of research material; Ethical considerations in research from a phenomenological perspective; Interpretation and analysis of phenomenologically oriented research for nursing and health care practice; Contribution of the phenomenological perspective in research to humanize health care delivery.

TEACHING STRATEGIES

1. Seminar.
2. Out of class: existential investigation, film viewing, biographies, autobiographies, fiction, poetry, and interviews, conversations.
3. In-class: phenomenological interpretation of out-of-class existential investigation.
4. Writing phenomenological narratives.
5. Interpreting meanings of narratives through dialogue.

EVALUATION METHODS

Weekly Annotated Bibliography Card	30%
Presentation of Research Article with Critique	25%
Presentation of Phenomenological Research	45%

REQUIRED TEXTS Munhall, P., & Oiler-Boyd, C. (1993). *Nursing research: A qualitative perspective.* New York: National League for Nursing

van Manen, M. (1990). *Researching lived experience: An action sensitive pedagogy.* New York: State University of New York.

Research journal readings.

Bibliography

Aamodt, A. (1986). Discovering the child's view of alopecia: Doing ethnography. In P. Munhall & c. Oiler (Eds.), *Nursing research: A qualitative perspective* (pp. 163-171). Norwalk, CT: Appleton-Century-Crofts.

Abdellah, F.G. (1969). The nature of nursing science. *Nursing Research, 8,* 390-393.

Allen, D., Benner, P., and Diekelmann, N. (1985). Three paradigms for nursing research: Methodological implications (chap. 3) in P. Chinn (Eds.), *Nursing Research Methodology Issues and Implementation.* Rockville, MD: Aspen.

Allen, D. (1991). Applying critical social theory to nursing education. In N. Greenleaf (Ed)., *Curriculum revolution: Redefining the student-teacher relationship.* New York: National League for Nursing.

Allen, D. (1985). Nursing research and social control: Alternative models of science that emphasize understanding and emancipation. *Image, 17,* 58-64.

Allen, M., & Jensen, L. (1990). Hermeneutical inquiry: Meaning and scope. *Western Journal of Nursing Research, 12*(2), 241-253.

American Nurses' Association Policy Statement (1980).

Annas, D.J., Glantz, L.H., & Katz, B.J. (1977). *Informed consent to human experimentation: The subject's dilemma.* Boston: Ballinger.

Atwood, D., Stolorow, R. (1984). *Structures of subjectivity.* New Jersey: Lawrence Erlbaum Associates. (pp. 47-53).

Baer, E. (1979). Philosophy provide the rationale for nursing's multiple research directions. *Image, 2,* 72-74.

Barthes. In *Saybrook Review* (1986). p. 383.

Bateson, M.C. (1990). *Composing a life.* New York: Plume Books, Penguin.

Beattie, A. (1989). *Picturing will.* New York: Random House. (pp. 53).

Belenky, M., Clinchy, B., Goldberg, N., & Taub, J. (1986). *Women's ways of knowing.* New York: Basic Books.

Bellah, R. (1981). The ethical aims of social inquiry. *Teachers College Record, 83*(1), 1-18.

Benner, P. (1985). Quality of life: A phenomenological perspective on explanation, prediction, and understanding in nursing science. *Advances in Nursing Science, 8*(1), 1-14.

Benner, P. (1983). Uncovering the knowledge embedded in clinical practice. *Image: The Journal of Nursing Scholarship, 19,* 21-34.

Benner, P., Wrubel, J. (1989). *The primacy of caring stress and coping in health and illness.* Menlo Park, CA: Addison-Wesley.

Benoliel, J. (1984). Advancing nursing science: Qualitative approaches. *Western Journal of Nursing Research, 6,* 1-8.

Bevis, E.O. (1988). Caring: A life force. In Leininger, M. (Ed.), *Caring: An essential human need.* (pp. 49-59). Detroit: Wayne State University Press.

Bronowski, J. (1965). *Science and human values.* (Rev. ed.). New York: Harper & Row.

Burns, N., & Grove, S. (1987). *The practice of nursing research: Conduct, critique and utilization.* Philadelphia: W.B. Saunders

Burns, N. (1989). Standards for qualitative research. *Nursing Science Quarterly, 2*(1), 44-52.

Carper, B.A. (1979). The ethics of caring. *Advances in Nursing Science, 1*(2), 11-19.

Carper, B. (1978). Fundamentals patterns of knowing. *Advanced Nursing Science, 13,* 23.

Chenitz, W.C., & Swanson, J.M. (1986). *From practice to grounded theory: Qualitative research in nursing.* Menlo Park, CA: Addison-Wesley.

Chinn, P. (1985). Debunking myths in nursing theory and research. *Image, 17,* 45-49.

Cohen, M. (1987). A historical overview of the phenomenological movement. *Image: The Journal of Nursing Scholarship, 19,* 31-34.

Colaizzi, P. (1973). *Reflection and research in psychology.* Dubuque: Kendall Hunt Publishing Co.

Colaizzi, P. (1978). Psychological research as the phenomenologist views it. In Valle and King (Eds.), *Existential phenomenological alternatives for psychology.* New York: Oxford University Press.

Connors, D. (1988). The continuum of the researcher—participant relationships: An analysis and critique. *Advances in Nursing Sciences, 10*(4), 32-42.

Cowling, W.R. (1986). Methods: A reflective model. In P. Chinn (Ed.), *Nursing research methodology: Issues and implementation.* Rockland, MD: Aspen.

Curtin, L. (1979). The nurse as advocate: A philosophical foundation for nursing. *Advances in Nursing Science, 8*(3).

Davis, A. (1973). The phenomenological approach in nursing research. In E. Garrison (Ed.), *Doctoral preparation for nurses* (pp. 212-228). San Francisco: University of California.

Dilthey, W. (1985). *Poetry and experience.* Selected Works, Vol. V, Princeton, NJ: Princeton University Press.

Dilthey, W. (1926). *Meaning in history.* London: Allen & Unwin.

Dilthey, W. (1987). *Introduction to the human sciences.* Toronto: Scholarly Book Services.

Dossey, L. (1982). *Space, time, and medicine.* Boulder, CO: Shambala.

Douglas, J.D. (1979). Living morality versus bureaucratic fist. In C.B. Klockars & F.W. O'Connor (Eds.), *Deviance and decency.* Beverly Hills, CA: Sage.

Dreyfus, H. (1972). *What computers can't do: A critique of artifical reason.* New York: Harper & Row.

Duke, P. & Hochman, G. (1992). *A brilliant madness: Living with manic-depressive illness.* New York: Bantam Books.

Dzurec, L. (1989). The necessity for and evolution of multiple paradigms for nursing research: A poststructural perspective. *Advances in Nursing Science, 11*(4), 69-77.

Estes, C.P. (1992). *Women who run with the wolves: Myths and stories of the wild woman archtype.* Ballentine Books.

Estroff, S.E., & Churchill, L.R. (1984). Comment (Ethical dilemmas). *Anthropology Newsletter, 25*(7).

Fawcett, J. The metaparadigm of nursing: Present status and future refinements. *Image, 19;* 16(3), 84-7.

Feyerabend, P.K. (1981). *Philosophical papers.* Vol. 1. Cambridge, England: Cambridge University Press.

Field, P.A., & Morse, J.M. (1985). *Nursing research: The application of qualitative approaches.* Rockville, MD: Aspen.

Fischer, C., & Wertz, F. (1979). Empirical phenomenological analysis of being criminally victimized. In A. Giorgi, A. Barton, & C. Maes (Eds.), *Duquesne studies in phenomenological psychology* (Vol. I). Pittsburgh: Duquesne University Press.

Forward, S. (1991). *Obsessive love.* New York: Bantam Books.

Gadamer, G.H., Sheed & Ward, Ltd. (1975). *Truth and method.* New York: Crossroad.

Freire, P. (1970). *Pedagogy of the oppressed.* New York, New York: Seabury Press.

Georgi, A. (1970). *Psychology as a human science: A phenomenological based approach.* New York: Harper & Row.

Giorgi, A. (1965). Phenomenology and experimental psychology, I. *Review of Existential Psychology and Psychiatry, 5*(1), pp. 37-50.

Glaser, B., & Strauss, A. (1967). *The discovery of grounded theory.* Chicago: Aldine.

Gould, S.J. (1984, August 12). Science and gender. *The New York Times Book Review.*

Greenson, J. (1993). *It's not what you're eating: It's what's eating you.*

Haase, J. (1987). Components of courage in chronically ill adolescents: A phenomenological study. *Advances in Nursing Science, 9,* 64-80.

Habermas, J. (1971). *Knowledge and human interests.* Boston, MA: Beacon.

Hardy, M.E. (1974). Theories: components, development, evaluation. *Nursing Research, 23,* 100-107.

Heidegger, M. (1971). *On the way to language.* New York: Harper & Row.

Heidegger, M. (1949). *Existence and being.* Chicago: Regnery.

Heidegger, M. (1962). *Being and time.* (Macquarrie & Robinson Trans). San Francisco: Harper & Row Publishers.

Hubell, S. (1993). *Broadsides from the other order: A bug of book.* New York: Random House.

Husserl, E. (1965). *Phenenomenology and the crisis of philosophy.* (Z. Lauer, Trans). New York: Harper & Row.

Hutchinson, S. (1986). Grounded theory: The method. In P. Munhall & C. Oiler (Eds.). *Nursing research: A qualitative perspective.* Norwalk, CT: Appleton-Century-Crofts.

Huxley, J.H. (1982). *Space, time and medicine.* Boulder, CO: Shambhala. (pp. 225).

Jacox, A. (1974). Theory construction in nursing: An overview. *Nursing Research, 23,* 4-13.

Kaplan, A. (1965). *The conduct of inquiry.* Scranton, PA: Chandler.

Kayson, S. (1993). *Girl, interrupted.* New York: Turtle Bay Books.

Kirk, J., & Miller, M. (1986). *Reliability and validity in qualitative research.* Newbury Park, CA: Sage.

Knafl, K., & Howard, M. (1986). Interpreting, reporting, and evaluating qualitative research. In P. Munhall & C. Oiler (Eds.), *Nursing research: A qualitative perspective.* Norwalk, CT: Appleton-Century-Crofts.

Kubler-Ross, E. (1969). *On death and dying.* New York: Macmillan.

Kuhn, T. S. (Ed.). (1970). *The structure of scientific revolutions.* Chicago: University of Chicago Press.

Kurtz, S. (1989). *The art of unknowing.* New Jersey: Aronson, Inc. (pp. 6-9).

Langer, M. (1989). *Marleau-Ponty's phenomenology of perception.* Tallahassee, FL: The Florida State University Press.

Laudan, L. (1977). *Progress and its problems: Toward a theory of scientific growth.* Berkeley, CA: University of California Press.

Leininger, M. (1985). *Qualitative research methods in nursing.* New York: Grune & Stratton.

Leininger, M. (1981). *Caring: An essential human need.* Thorofare, NJ: Charles B. Slack.

Light, R., & Pillemer, D. (1982). Numbers and narrative: Combining their strengths in research reviews. *Harvard Education Review, 52*(1), 1-23.

Lincoln, Y., & Guba, E. (1985). *Nauralistic inquiry.* Newbury Park, CA: Sage.

Ludemann, R. (1979). The paradoxical nature of nursing research. *Image, 2,* 2-8.

Lynch-Sauer, J. (1985). Using phenomenological research to study nursing phenomena. In M. Leininger (Ed.), *Qualitative research methods in nursing* (pp. 93-107). Orlando, FL: Grune & Stratton.

MacPherson, K. (1983). Feminist methods: A new paradigm for nursing research. *Advances in Nursing Service, 5,* 17-25.

Marquez, G.G. (1970). *One hundred years of solitude.* New York: Harper & Row.

McPhee, J. (1989). *The control of nature.* New York: Farrer, Straus and Girioux. (pp. 11).

Meleis, A.P. (1986). The development and domain concepts. In P. Moccia (Eds.), *New approaches to theory development.* New York: National League for Nursing.

Meleis, A. (1985). *Theoretical nursing: Development and progress.* Philadelphia: Lippincott.

Merleau-Ponty, M. (1956). *What is phenomenology?* Cross Currents, 6, 59-70.

Merleau-Ponty, M. (1964). *The primary of perception.* (J. Edie, Trans.). Evanston, IL: Northwestern University Press.

Merleau-Ponty, M. (1962). *Phenomenology of perception.* (C. Smith, Trans). New York: Humanities Press.

Miles, M., & Huberman, A. (1984). *Qualitative data analysis: A sourcebook of new methods.* Newbury Park, CA: Sage

Moccia, P. (1986). Theory development and nursing practice: A synposis of a study of the theory-practice diabetic. In Moccia, P., ed., *New approaches to theory development.* New York: National League for Nursing.

Moccia, P. (1988). A critique of compromise: Beyond the methods debate. *Advances in Nursing Science, 10*(4), 1-9.

Moccia, P. (Ed.). (1986). *New approaches in theory development.* New York: National League for Nursing.

Moccia, P. (1986a). The theory-practice dialectic. In P. Moccia, (Ed.), *New approaches to theory developement.* New York: National League for Nursing.

Moccia, P. (1986b). The dialectic as method. In P. Chinn (Ed.). *Nursing research methodology: Issues and implementation.* Rockland, MD: Aspen.

Morgan, G. (1983). *Beyond method.* Beverly Hills, CA: Sage.

Morse, J. (1988). Commentaries on special issue. *Western Journal of Nursing Research, 10*(2), 213-216.

Morse, J. (1991). *Qualitative nursing research: A contemporary dialogue.* Newbury Park: Sage Publications.

Munhall, P. (1992). Holding the Mississippi River in place and other implications for qualitative research. *Nursing Outlook, 40*(6), 257-262.

Munhall, P. & Oiler, C. (1986). *Nursing research: A qualitative perspective.* Norwalk, CT: Appleton-Century-Crofts.

Munhall, P. (1982). Nursing philosophy and nursing research. In apposition or opposition. *Nursing Research, 31,* 176-181.

Munhall, P.L. (1989). Philosophical ponderings on qualitative research methods in nursing. *Nursing Science Quarterly,* 20-28.

Munhall, P., & Oiler, C. (1987). Human values in nursing: Esthetic expressions. Poster presentation at the American Nurses Association, Council of Nurse Researchers International Nursing Research Conference, Washington, D.C.

Munhall, P. (1988). Ethical considerations in qualitative research. *Western Journal of Nursing Research, 10*(2), 150-162.

Nesbitt, R. (1976). *Sociology as an art form.* New York: Oxford University.

Newman, M., Sime, A., & Cocoran-Perry. (1991). The focus of the discipline of nursing. *Advances in Nursing Science, 14*(1), 1-5.

Newman, M.A. (1979). *Theory development in nursing.* Philadelphia: Davis.

Newman, M.A. (1986). *Health as expanding consciousness.* St. Louis, MO: Mosby.

Newman, M.A. (1983). Editorial. *Advances in Nursing Science, 5,* X-XI.

Noble, M. (1985). Written informed consent: closing the door to clinical research. *Nusing Outlook, 33*(6), 292-293.

Norris, C. (1982). *Concept clarification in nursing.* Rockville, MD: Aspen.

Oberst, M. (1985). Another look at informed consent. *Nursing Outlook, 33*(6), 294-295.

Oiler, C. (1982). The phenomenological approach in nursing research. *Nursing Research, 31*(3), 178-181.

Oiler, C. (1986a). In P. Munhall & C. Oiler (Eds.) *Nursing research: A qualitative perspective.* Norwalk, CT: Appleton-Century-Crofts.

Oiler, B.C. (1988). Phenomenology: A foundation for nursing curriculum. In National League for Nursing, *Curriculum revolution: Mandate for change.* New York: National League for Nursing.

Oiler, C. (1986b). Qualitative methods: Phenomenology. In P. Moccia (Ed.). *New approaches to theory development.* New York: National League for Nursing.

Omery, A. (1983). Phenomenology: A method for nursing reearch. *Advances in Nursing Science, 5,* 178-181.

Parse, R., Coyne, A., & Smith, M. (1985). *Nursing research: Qualitative methods.* Bowie, MD: Brady Communications Company

Parse, R.R. (1987). *Nursing science: Major paradigms, theories, and critiques.* Philadelphia: Saunders.

Parse, R.R. (1981). *Man-living-health: A theory of nursing.* New York: Wiley.

Parse, R. (1990). Parse's research methodology with an illustration of the lived experience of hope. *Nursing Science Quarterly, 3*(1), 9-17.

Paterson & Zderad. (1976). *Humanistic nursing.* New York: Wiley. Reprinted 1988. New York: National League for Nursing.

Patient Self Determination Act. (1991). Amnibus Budget Reconcilliation Act of 1990. (OBRA-90).

Polkinghorne, D. (1983). *Methodology for the human sciences.* Albany: SUNY Press.

Postman, N. (1992). *Technopoly.* New York: Alfred A. Knopf.

Psathas, G. (1973). *Phenomenological sociology: Issues and applications.* New York: John Wiley & Sons.

Punch, M. (1986). *The politics of ethics of fieldwork.* Beverly Hills, CA: Sage.

Ray, M. (1990). Phenomenological method for nursing research. In Chaska, H. (Ed.), *The nursing profession: Turning points.* Orlando, FL: Grune & Stratton

Reeder, F. (1987). The phenomenological movement. *Image, 19,* 150-152.

Relke, R. (1977). *Possibility of being.* New York: A New Directions Book.

Ricoeur, P., Thompson, J. (1983). *Hermeneutics and the human sciences.* London, England: Cambridge University Press.

Rock, P. (1979). *The making of symbolic interactionism.* London: Macmillan.

Rogers, M.E. (1970). *An introduction to the theoretical basis of nursing.* Philadelphia, PA: Davis.

Rogers, M.E. (1986). Science of unitary human beings. In V. Malinski (Ed.). *Explorations on Matha Rogers' science of unitary human beings.* Norwalk, CT: Appleton-Century-Crofts.

Rorty, R. (1990, December 2). Richard Porty: Philosopher. *New York Times Magazine.*

Sacks, O. (1990). *The man who mistook his wife for a hat.* New York: Harper Perennial.

Sanday, P. (1983). The ethnographic paradigm. In Van Manen (Ed.), *Qualitative methodology.* (pp. 19-35). Beverly Hills, CA: Sage.

Sandelowski, H. (1986). The problem of rigor in qualitative research. *Advances in Nursing Science, 8*(3), 27-31.

Sarter, B. (1988a). *The stream of becoming: A study of Martha Rogers' theory.* New York: National League for Nursing.

Sarter, B. (19881). Philosophical sources of nursing theory. *Nursing Science Quarterly, 1,* 52-59.

Sartre, J.P. (1966). *Being and nothingness.* New York: Washington Square Press.

Schutz, A. (1970). In H. Wagner (Ed.). *On phenomenology and social relations.* Chicago: University of Chicago Press.

Schutz, A. (1973). *Collected papers I: The problem of social reality.* (M. Natanson, Ed.). The Hague, Netherlands: Martinus Nijhoff.

Sederbar, B. (1989). *Politics of meaning.* Tucson, AZ: The Arizona University Press.

Sheehy, G. (1992). *The silent passage: Menopause.* New York: Random House.

Silva, M. (1977). Philosophy, science, theory: Interrelationships and implications for nursing research. *Image, 9,* 59-63.

Silva, M., & Rothbart, D. (1984, January). An analysis of changing trends in philosophies of science on nursing theory development and testing. *Advances in Nursing Science, 6*(2).

Silva, M. & Rothbart. (1984). Philosophies of science on nursing theory: Development and testing. *Advances in Nursing Science, 6,* 1-13.

Smiley, J. (1989). *Ordinary love and good will.* New York: Random House. (pp. 120).

Spiegelberg, H. (1982). *The phenomenological movement.* The Hague: Martinus Nijhoff.

Spiegelberg, H. (1975). *Doing phenomenology.* The Hague, Netherlands: Martinus Nijhoff.

Spradley, J. (1980). *Participant observation.* New York: Holt, Rinhart & Winston.

Stern, P. (1980). Grounded theory methodology: Its use and processes. *Image, 12,* 20-23.

Swanson, J., & chenitz, C. (1982). Why qualitative research in nursing? *Nursing Outlook, 30,* 241-245.

Thompson, J.B. (1984). *Studies in the theory of ideology.* Berkeley, CA: University of California Press.

Tinkle, M., & Beaton, J. (1983). Toward a new view of science: Implications for nursing research. *Advances in Nursing Science, 5,* 27–36.

Tripp-Reimer, T., & Cohen, M. Z. (1989). Funding strategies for qualitative research. In J. M. Morse (Ed.), *Qualitative nursing research: A contemporary dialogue* (pp. 225–238). Rockville, MD: Aspen.

U.S. Department of Health and Human Services. (1991). *Healthy People Year 2000.* Washington: U.S. Department of Health and Human Services.

van Kaam, A. (1969). *Existential foundations of psychology.* New York: Doubleday.

van Manen, M. (1990). *Researching the lived experience.* Ontario, Canada: State University of New York Press.

van Manen, M. (1984b). Practicing phenomenological writing. *Phenomenology & pedagogy, 2*(1), 36–69.

van Kaam, A. (1959). Phenomenal analysis: Exemplified by a study of the experience of "really feeling understood." *Journal of Individual Psychology, 15,* 66–72.

van Manen, M. (1984a). *"Doing" phenomenological research and writing: An introduction.* (Curriculum Praxis Monograph No. 7). Edmonton, Canada: University of Alberta.

Wagner, H. (1983). *Phenomenology of consciousness and sociology of the life-world.* Edmonton, Alberta: The University of Alberta Press.

Warwick, D.P. (1982). Tearsome trade: Means and ends in social research. In M. Bulmer (Ed.), *social research ethics.* London: Macmillan.

Watson, J. (1981). Nursing's scientific quest. *Nursing Outlook, 29*(7), 413–416.

Watson, J. (1988, Fall). New dimensions of human caring theory. *Nursing Science Quarterly,* 175–181.

Watson, J. (1979). *Nursing: The philosophy and science of caring.* Boston: Little. Brown.

Watson, J. (1985). *Nursing: Human science and human care: A theory of nursing.* Norwal, CT: Appleton-Century-Crofts.

Wilson, L., & Fitzpatrick, J. (1984). Dialectic thinking as a means of understanding systems in development: Relevance to Roger's principles. *Advances in Nursing Service, 6*(2), 41.

Wilson, H.S. (1985). *Research in Nursing.* Menlo Park, CA: Addison-Wesley.

Wolfe, T. (1987). *The bonfire of the vanities.* Giroux, New York: Farrar, Strauss.

Yalon, I.D. (1992). *When Nietzsche wept.* Basic Books.

Index

321